Imagining Health

IMAGINING HEALTH

Medicine, Social Protest, and Modern American Literature

IRA HALPERN

University of Massachusetts Press
AMHERST AND BOSTON

Copyright © 2026 by University of Massachusetts Press
All rights reserved.
Printed in the United States of America

ISBN 978-1-62534-911-8 (paper); 912-5 (hardcover)

Designed by Deste Relyea
Set in Minion Pro and Bodoni
Printed and bound by Books International, Inc.

Cover design by adam b. bohannon

Library of Congress Cataloging-in-Publication Data

Names: Halpern, Ira, 1994– author
Title: Imagining health : medicine, social protest, and modern American literature / Ira Halpern.
Description: Amherst : University of Massachusetts Press, 2026. | Includes bibliographical references and index. | Identifiers: LCCN 2025017598 (print) | LCCN 2025017599 (ebook) | ISBN 9781625349118 paperback | ISBN 9781625349125 hardcover | ISBN 9781685751920 ebook | ISBN 9781685751937 epub
Subjects: LCSH: Medicine in literature | Progressivism in literature | Social movements in literature | American literature—20th century—History and criticism | LCGFT: Literary criticism
Classification: LCC PS228.M43 H35 2026 (print) | LCC PS228.M43 (ebook)
LC record available at https://lccn.loc.gov/2025017598
LC ebook record available at https://lccn.loc.gov/2025017599

British Library Cataloguing-in-Publication Data
A catalog record for this book is available from the British Library.

The authorized representative in the EU for product safety and compliance is Mare-Nostrum Group.
Email: gpsr@mare-nostrum.co.uk
Physical address: Mare-Nostrum Group B.V., Mauritskade 21D,
1091 GC Amsterdam, The Netherlands

For my parents

Contents

Acknowledgments

ix

INTRODUCTION

1

CHAPTER ONE
The Cost of Care

13

CHAPTER TWO
Professional Medicine and Racial Protest

36

CHAPTER THREE
Sexual Health and Women's Rights

74

CHAPTER FOUR
Disability, Euthanasia, Survival

107

CODA

130

Archival Collections

139

Notes

141

Index

159

Acknowledgments

Writing *Imagining Health* has been both a solitary and a collective experience. Throughout the process of doing so, I have been tremendously fortunate to receive generous feedback and support from many peers, colleagues, friends, and family.

Imagining Health first took shape at The University of Toronto's Department of English, where I completed my PhD; there, Michael Cobb, Naomi Morgenstern, Dana Seitler, Paul Downes, Andrea Most, Andrea Charise, and Randy Boyagoda, among others, offered advice and inspiration that profoundly influenced this book.

At The University of Notre Dame, where I served as a Postdoctoral Fellow at the John J. Reilly Center for Science, Technology, and Values, Robert Goulding, Anna Geltzer, Vania Smith-Oka, Margaret Meserve, Ijeoma Kola, and Katharine McCabe were all a delight to work with, and provided crucial input. At Notre Dame, Korey Garibaldi, Jason Ruiz, Sophie White, Sara Marcus, and Matthew Kilbane provided helpful insights as well. In addition, I enjoyed and greatly benefited from discussing some of *Imagining Health*'s material with Notre Dame students enrolled in "Health, Medicine, and American Literature" and "Health, Medicine, and American Culture."

At Northeastern University, I have been a Postdoctoral Fellow with the Department of English, funded by the Social Sciences and Humanities Research Council of Canada, and within that context, it has been wonderful to have benefited from Sari Altschuler's expertise in literature and medicine.

At The College of New Jersey, as a Visiting Assistant Professor of English and the Medical Humanities, I have had the tremendous pleasure of working with both faculty and students as I completed this book. I received invaluable comments from David Blake on the entire book. More generally, it has a been a pleasure to work with faculty both within and beyond the English Department at TCNJ. I am especially grateful for advice and guidance about *Imagining Health* from Samira Abdur-Rahman, Michele Lise Tarter, and Felicia Jean Steele. Michelle Ordini's support has been very helpful. In addition, discussions with students at TCNJ across a range of courses in American literature and the medical humanities—including "Medical

Memoir," "Health Care Politics," and "Literature of the United States"—have been critical to this book's development.

For conversation, encouragement, and conference opportunities, I am fortunate to have benefited from a range of other interlocutors, colleagues, and friends. In terms of the development of *Imagining Health* in particular, I owe thanks to Priscilla Wald, Joanna Krongold, Joan Judge, Miya Shaffer, Shanon Fitzpatrick, Ela Lichtblau, Rio Hartwell, Oonagh Devitt Tremblay, Stephanie Redekop, Maya Waitzer, Lisa Diedrich, Stephanie Browner, Don James McLaughlin, Vic Evangelista, Phil Barrish, Daniel Sterlin-Altman, Saj Soomal, and the Starkmans.

I benefited from presenting and discussing material from this book at conferences including the Modern Language Association of America (MLA) Annual Convention, the Health Humanities Consortium, the American Literature Association, the American Studies Association, the Northeast Popular Culture Association, and the Northeast Modern Language Association.

To the archivists and librarians across Canada and the US with whom I have consulted, I am grateful for helping make this book possible.

The editorial team at the University of Massachusetts Press has been a joy to work with. Brian Halley has been an incredibly supportive editor and has helped tremendously with the publishing process. Ben Kimball, Chelsey Harris, Sally Nichols, and Mary Dougherty have also been wonderful to work with. I am appreciative of Amber Williams' copyedits. In addition, I am deeply grateful for the invaluable feedback I received from the manuscript's anonymous peer reviewers solicited by the press.

Material from a version of chapter 1 appeared in *American Literature*; I am grateful to its editors for accepting my work to be published there at an early stage in the development of *Imagining Health* and for permission to publish a version of it here.

Finally, I have benefited from the support of my entire family. I am so grateful for the support of my parents and step-parents, Lesley and Mark, and Martin and Karen. I owe thanks to my siblings, Simone and Rebecca, and to Sheara and Shawn. I owe thanks to my cousins, especially Rachel, who provided feedback on some chapters, and my aunts and uncles, including Elliott and Susanne, Peter and Paula, and Caroline and Joe. I owe thanks to my grandparents, Esther and Stan.

And I am grateful for Niko.

Imagining Health

Introduction

AS US MEDICINE BECAME increasingly professionalized around the turn of the twentieth century, it gained unprecedented diagnostic and therapeutic power. But while acknowledging the undeniable value of the medical establishment, modern fiction writers both reimagined and actively transformed the politics of care. As the medical establishment developed at the end of the nineteenth century, it began to resemble what exists today. Technologies proliferated, specializations expanded, and medical education became standardized. Yet, alongside these developments, many patients and populations struggled to access and benefit from the highest levels of care. Moving into the twentieth century, literary writers confronting social ills within their work offered critiques of modern medicine and portrayed what they viewed as better alternatives. As I argue, by interweaving scenes of professional medicine with commitments to the social-protest movements and ideas rippling through the nation, American fiction writers positioned the right to health as a key aim of progressive politics. These authors—among them Robert Herrick, Wallace Thurman, A. L. Furman, Frank Slaughter, Charles Chesnutt, Walter White, Ralph Ellison, Charlotte Perkins Gilman, Upton Sinclair, Stephen Crane, Edith Wharton, and Dalton Trumbo—anchored their understandings of health to broad currents of reform and efforts at social transformation, including counter-capitalist critiques, racial protest, women's rights, and an incipient form of disability justice. Their medical commentary both informed and was influenced by their fiction. Throughout their lives, they directly engaged with professional and institutional forms of medical care, reflecting upon their experiences with physicians and hospitals, reading and commenting on medical publications, joining organizations active in health reform, and participating in discussions about public health. Throughout their work, these authors took a distinctly political approach to sickness, injury, and debilitation, and in response to their encounters with these experiences, they called for collective social change.

Their fiction was published at a time in which the medical professions were held in a particularly high regard. In and around the early twentieth century, a faith in professional authority swept through American culture, as individuals came to place an unprecedented trust in the professional expertise of select citizens from the middle-classes, including reformers and altruists, in part emerging from their perceived capacity to resolve social problems. Social workers, librarians, teachers, lawyers, journalists, and writers were all part of this increasingly powerful professional class. But in attaining widespread respect, prestige, and status, the medical professions, in no small part because of the explanatory power of science upon which their expertise rested, did so particularly successfully.[1] American authors in this period often recognized the newfound promise of medical innovations and authority even as they took a critical look at modern medicine. Because of the various scientific, technological, and professional developments unfolding in the medical establishment at the time in which they were writing, these authors could not abandon or entirely reject modern medicine. Instead, they called for it to be transformed and reconfigured to advance a progressive politics of care.

To be sure, there are long traditions of health reform and medical critique that have entailed insisting on complete alternatives to conventional professional medicine. In the early to mid-nineteenth century, many prominent critiques of medicine were based on significant suspicion of medical authority—what Paul Starr calls "therapeutic nihilism"[2]—often bound up in a populist, anti-elitist sensibility that was skeptical of scientific expertise. Reformers, informal healers, and literary writers sought to empower everyday Americans to take charge of their health rather than consult professional experts. For much of the eighteenth and nineteenth centuries, physicians' work had lacked formal structure, and options for healing, as Nancy Tomes notes, were characterized by an "abundance of care, none of it any good,"[3] which led many citizens, and even doctors, to question professional medical authority. The early American spirit of anti-professional critique is apparent in the title of Scottish-born Virginian doctor John Tennent's widely reprinted pamphlet *Every Man His Own Doctor* (1734),[4] which proposed home remedies for a range of diseases above professional expertise and a recourse to medical jargon. In line with this sentiment, a popular health movement, governed by Jacksonian principles, swept through America. John C. Gunn published a home medical guide in 1830 that emphasized "principles of common sense" in medical matters: he promised that if everyday Americans followed his advice on self-medication, water and mineral treatments, medicinal herbs, exercise, and temperance they would not need advice from physicians.[5] The celebrated poet Walt Whitman similarly recommended in *Manly Health and Training* (1858), published under the pseudonym Mose Velsor, that American men should preserve their physical and psychological health through diet, exercise, and grooming, instead of consulting dubious doctors. According to Whitman, medical expertise was often superfluous. Instead, Whitman privileged "common reason" noting, "generally speaking, the benefit of medicine, or medical advice is very much overrated. Nature's medicines are simple food, nursing, air, rest, cheerful encouragement, and the like." Whitman complained that the art of the physician could be "vague, and affords an easy cover to ignorance and quackery," adding that the "land is too full of poisonous medicines and incompetent doctors—the less you have to do with them the better."[6] A deep suspicion of medical professionalization pervaded American culture, fueled by a weariness about its increasingly elite status, making the notion that everyone should be their "own doctor" continually appealing. In fact, the health of the nation and the power of everyday citizens over their bodies and minds seemed to depend on it.

Many nineteenth-century Americans became enthralled by alternative health crusades, especially those that emphasized laypeople's power to transform themselves. Health reform movements were predicated on hygienic ideology, which held that personal hygiene was critical to individuals' moral progress. They deemed it essential to attend to the "laws of nature" concerning dress, exercise, and diet, even when those laws ran counter to more established scientific opinion.[7] For instance, Thomsonianism, promulgated by Samuel Thomson, a self-taught botanist, advocated for herbal remedies to treat a range of ailments. Thomson appealed to anti-elitist sensibilities. As noted in a preface "written by a friend" to his *New Guide to Health* in "plain language," doctors were deliberately keeping people "ignorant of every thing of importance in medicine, by its being kept in a dead language, for which there can be no good reason given. . . ." In this view, doctors had so much "influence in society, and manage[d] their affairs with so much art for their own profit and praise" that "the common people" were deprived of the knowledge they needed.[8] Another popular healing modality, homeopathy—which took hold when Hans Burch Gram introduced it to America in the early nineteenth century—was premised on the notion that "like cures like," the theory that diluting a substance causing disease in healthy people could cure similar symptoms in sick people. Presbyterian minister Sylvester Graham likewise presented challenges to conventional medical authority by prescribing a strict dietary regimen as a path toward health; in time, his graham cracker became an affordable household staple. In addition, Mary Sargeant Gove Nichols and her husband developed hydrotherapy, emphasizing baths, liberal water consumption, exercise, and fresh air. Nichols combined the water cure with a commitment to marriage reform and "free love," training patients in her New York City water-cure boarding house not only in bathing but also in toppling patriarchy and the strictures of marriage.[9] Proponents of self-care and alternative therapies were responding to harsh medical realities, advocating gentler substitutes for the invasive therapeutics of the conventional, "regular" profession such as bleeding and purging, while also aligning with agendas that reflected their political principles.

Resonating with the political impulses behind earlier reform movements that sought to democratize health and challenge hegemonic forms of medical authority, the generations of writers whom I focus on here, publishing in and around the early to mid-twentieth century, also encountered the rapid professionalization and institutionalization of medicine, and they had to account for its tremendous power. In response, they centered the conventional medical establishment in their critiques while simultaneously privileging its reform and radical transformation.

Around the mid-nineteenth through the turn of the twentieth century, US medical care became increasingly systemized and powerful. These years saw various scientific and technological innovations that contributed to medicine's bolstered power. Central to this development was the Civil War, which greatly accelerated the expansion of US hospitals. Although medical professionals were initially unprepared for the war's taxing demands, during it they went on to refine dissection techniques, conduct microscopic analyses, study diseases such as gangrene, and collect patient data, publishing their findings in journals and implementing sanitary measures, including the use of disinfectants, to reduce contagion.

The late nineteenth century witnessed a reaction against the excessive rationalism of nineteenth-century medicine and heroic therapies as they gave way to scientific empiricism. American physicians studied at universities in Paris, as well as Vienna, and Berlin, and brought back to the United States the latest clinical methods. The final quarter of the nineteenth century witnessed a blossoming of physiology, pathology, and laboratory science. The development of modern medicine was largely enabled by the consolidation of the germ theory of disease over the 1860s through the 1880s, in the wake of experiments conducted by Louis Pasteur and Robert Koch. While outbreaks of cholera in nineteenth-century America undermined physicians' cultural authority, by the mid-twentieth century, physicians had brought under control diseases such as smallpox, tuberculosis, and diphtheria. As a result, medical care was becoming a life-saving resource, yielding notable municipal and national benefits. Antisepsis, anesthetics, and X-rays made surgeries safer and more successful, while improvements in living standards, along with philanthropic and government investments in hospitals, medical education, and research, fostered a newfound confidence in scientific medicine.

Moving into the twentieth century, medical education and licensing were increasingly standardized, with an increasing emphasis placed on science and university-affiliated research, and the closing down of small, for-profit medical schools. Admission to medical schools became more competitive and began to require more rigorous pre-medical coursework as prerequisites. Harvard University developed laboratory courses alongside traditional research, and Johns Hopkins emphasized practical hospital experience in medical training, becoming a model for other medical schools across the nation. The 1870s saw the creation of the Association of American Medical Colleges which helped develop a curricula shared by many US medical schools. As medical work became increasingly formalized, membership within the American Medical Association, which had been established in 1847, expanded from approximately 8,000 in 1900 to 70,000 members in 1910, and the AMA established the Council on Medical Education to improve licensure standards. Physicians participated in the establishment of state and local boards of health that raised standards of care; by the early 1900s, most states had operationalized medical licensing boards.[10]

Attempts at grappling with the transformation toward a more widely embraced professionalized system of medical care can be seen in American literary culture, as writers closely observed medical developments and sought to influence popular opinion on them. Novelist and social critic Mark Twain, skeptical of traditional medicine, experimented throughout the nineteenth century with and advocated for alternative therapies, but in the early twentieth century, his views were coming to seem outmoded. He sought to empower individuals with the autonomy to choose the kind of medical expertise of which they would avail themselves.[11] Consider, for instance, Twain's 1901 "Remarks on Osteopathy" that he delivered before a Committee on Public Health in the New York General Assembly in Albany in response to the Seymour Bill to license osteopaths in the state of New York. Twain talked about wanting to hold on to his "free will" in medical matters. He noted his mother had raised him with the cold-water cure, even as he acknowledged that the "ministering angel with the pills" was sometimes called upon. But by the early twentieth century, it was difficult to wholly discredit the conventional medical professions.[12] In fact, Twain's stance drew intense criticism. His intent to defend liberty over the body sounded not only antiquated but downright dangerous. For instance, Twain was dismissed by a doctor, Robert Morris, as a humorist who should not be commenting on such serious matters. "Mark Twain," Morris quipped, "may come to us with jokes, but we are here dealing with life and death." This sentiment resounded in the wider public, with a *Times* article referring to Twain as a "public enemy."[13]

The critique of even Twain's qualified medical skepticism at the turn of the twentieth century encapsulates a broader cultural shift toward the recognition of conventional medicine's many benefits. By the time physician-poet William Carlos Williams wrote his 1951 autobiography, he articulated a broader consensus in American life about the critical importance of modern medicine: "By and large we couldn't live in the world today were it not for the medical profession . . . We'd plain die, masses of us, tomorrow, if medical techniques were not kept up no matter what our fractional beliefs might be."[14] Optimism in medicine over the coming decades found expression in popular culture. These years saw what Christopher R. Cashman calls the "myth of the medical researcher hero," exemplified by Paul de Kruif's *Microbe Hunters* (1926), which celebrated major achievements in science for a popular audience; Sinclair Lewis's *Arrowsmith* (1925), which valorized the pursuit of scientific research through the career of its physician protagonist; and Frederick Schiller Faust's *Dr. Kildare* series of the 1930s and 1940s which centered on a protagonist's professional and personal successes in the medical field.[15]

The professionalization and institutionalization of medicine led to an acceptance of the fundamental basis of its expertise, and some have called the period of time in and around the mid-twentieth century the "golden age" of American medicine.[16] But while this characterization accurately calls attention to the scientific and professional developments that dramatically increased medicine's effectiveness in this era, it obscures the medical injustices that authors exposed and critiqued as they drew conceptual connections between medical care and major currents of social protest. As they envisioned expanding access to medical care, combating medical violence, and challenging stigmas associated with illness, injury, and disability, they aimed to enact ambitious transformations of national significance. They did not portray changes to the medical system as merely reflective of progressive movements, but they recognized that medical interventions were co-constitutive of some of the era's most transformative visions of social and political change.

In this period, ideas about the constitution of a healthy nation offered within the pages of American fiction were rapidly evolving and expanding. As Joan Burbick has shown, nineteenth-century American writers such as Walt Whitman, Edgar Allan Poe, Herman Melville, Oliver Wendell Holmes Sr., and Emily Dickinson had often used the rhetoric of national health to gauge the republic's functioning, yet typically with reference to a white, middle-class, and able-bodied body politic. As Josh Doty notes in a discussion of literary representations of health and the body in the nineteenth century, antebellum health reform efforts, including dietary regimens, temperance, hydrotherapy, and physiological education, were "typically white, male, middle-class enterprises that served white, male, middle-class priorities." While there were exceptions to this homogeneity even in the early nineteenth century, the authors whom I discuss, of later generations, offered a more wide-ranging set of perspectives, foregrounding the intersections of health with various forms of social oppression and political change.[17]

Their work, which renders the politics of health and medicine realistically, provokes interpretations attentive to concrete, material conditions shaping physical and psychological suffering. As such, in discussing their fiction, I do not read for health as a metaphor, which would mean taking up sickness, injury, and debility as figurations of other social ills. I take to heart Susan Sontag's warning that metaphors of illness and health often lead to the stigmatization of the unhealthy or the romanticization of suffering.[18] They can also detract attention from the literal experience of health itself, which merits sustained attention in its own right. Alternatively, realistic literature about medicine, though taking fictional form, often demystifies experiences of ill-health, pointing to its tangible social causes and consequences. In attending to this, my critical approach resonates with Sander Gilman's emphasis on representations of the unavoidable realities suffering. While Gilman shows how suffering is represented in and mediated by literary and visual culture, he notes that "those who deny the reality of the experience of disease marginalize and exclude the ill from their own world. . . . For the palpable signs of illness, the pain and suffering of the patient, cannot be simply dismissed as a social construction. . . ."[19] In the literary works discussed here, disease and injury appear not as social or cultural constructions but as concrete realities that serve as relays into lived experiences.

Social realism was an especially suitable genre for addressing these experiences. Realism and medicine have been considered as deeply entangled in that they both have focused, as Lawrence Rothfield demonstrates, on offering accurate visions of everyday life with expert precision, cultivating a "professional exactitude . . . useful to novelists when new conditions of the marketplace enabled writers to picture themselves as self-sufficient professions."[20] The diagnostic gaze fascinated realists over the mid-nineteenth and early twentieth centuries as they grappled with embodied and psychologically felt experiences of health and care. In addition to the sense in which a distinctly professional aesthetic dovetailed with concepts of medical expertise and objectivity, realism is also critical to my analysis because of its emphasis on social problems. Realistic fiction writers portrayed everyday life in great detail, focusing on the lives of not only the middle classes but also the socially disempowered. While certain forms of high literary realism could have an anti-didactic thrust, social realism often attempted to teach readers lessons about social problems. The authors discussed here rendered health realistically and imagined how a collective politics of health could become advanced through specific medical practices and policies. As Amanda Claybaugh shows, social realism expanded the purview of literary representation to incorporate attention to previously neglected issues such as poverty, slums, enslavement, labor, politics, dirt, and—as is especially relevant for my purposes here—disease, which, for these writers, has profoundly shaped and been shaped by these other kinds of social concerns.[21]

Investigating works that foreground the politics of medical care, in each chapter of *Imagining Health* I examine a realistic literary response to a specific juncture in which medical developments converged with progressive social movements that authors both recognized and contributed to as they sought to remake American health. In chapter 1, I examine early literary depictions of the medical economy, showing how fiction has helped envision publicly funded alternatives to a largely private medical system. Although the US private medical system is central to twentieth-century political debates, it has been largely neglected in literary and cultural studies. Yet novels from the early to mid-twentieth century mounted incisive critiques of that system. Robert Herrick's *The Healer* (1911) depicts a doctor who initially provides free care in the wilderness but then confronts the inflated costs of urban medicine, as Herrick renders emerging aspirations and anxieties about socialist medicine. Wallace Thurman and A. L. Furman's *The Interne* (1932) reveals corruption at a thinly fictionalized hospital on New York's Blackwell's Island during the Depression, illustrating the compromised state of public medical care and critiquing the logic of privatization that leads to dysfunctionality within public systems. Frank Slaughter's *That None Should Die* (1941), though weary of completely government-controlled medicine, advocates for expanded national insurance as a critical step toward health reform. Although these novels were published at different points in US medicine's evolution, all argue not only for an ethics of charity and compassion at the level of the individual doctor-patient encounter but for a robust publicly funded medical system more broadly.

Chapter 2 turns to the intersections of professional medical care and racial protest. Racial health inequities have been produced by segregation, and medical violence, as well as injurious, even lethal forms of neglect. In this chapter, I foreground fiction that responded to these problems by envisioning reclaimed and reimagined forms of medical authority. In *The Marrow of Tradition* (1901), Charles Chesnutt critiques the politics of cross-racial care and underscores the potential for medical professionals to improve Black communities' health. Years later, Walter White's collaboration with the NAACP to desegregate medicine coalesced with the impetus behind his novel *The Fire in the Flint* (1924), which points to entrenched racism in

US medical care and calls for alternatives rooted in the civic and political potential of medical work. Similarly, Ralph Ellison's *Invisible Man* (1952) can be interpreted in part as a critique of racial health inequities, particularly in mental health, in ways that were profoundly shaped by Ellison's involvement with the Lafargue Clinic in Harlem. Through their fiction, Chesnutt, White, and Ellison emphasized the importance of Black representation within the medical professions alongside the need for much broader social transformations.

Chapter 3 focuses on Charlotte Perkins Gilman and Upton Sinclair, tracing their contributions to the intertwined efforts of women's rights and sexual health advocacy. I examine Gilman's dialogue with a range of physicians, revealing how she adapted medical theories intended to eradicate venereal diseases in ways that furthered women's autonomy. Alongside her reform work, this dynamic plays out in her novel *The Crux* (1910) and in her short fiction. However, Gilman endorsed eugenic principles, which shaped her sexual-health politics and foreclosed much of the potential of her advocacy. Following the discussion of Gilman, I consider Upton Sinclair's public health–oriented writing and especially his overlooked novel *Sylvia's Marriage* (1914), which centers on women's sexual health and bodily autonomy. Sinclair too, however, was complicit in eugenics. Both Gilman and Sinclair held that implementing sexual-health education, reforming laws, and challenging social conventions around sexuality were essential to advancing women's health, as they resisted the patriarchal inflection of conventional love plots, medical secrecy, and double standards shaping sexual health discourse. At the same time, the disciplinary dimensions of their work present a fraught genealogy of sexual health reform that was both progressive and flawed.

Chapter 4 investigates critical responses to arguments for euthanasia. Advocates for euthanasia made claims to protect national health, but they did so by excluding disabled patients and populations from this vision and, in fact, they actively sought to eliminate disability from the social body. In response, fiction writers criticized and unsettled euthanasia arguments, insisting instead on respect for the wishes of disabled patients and valuing their survival. Stephen Crane, Edith Wharton, and Dalton Trumbo each critiqued the notion that disabled lives could lack inherent value. Even those advocating a right to die recognized how this discourse could shift into a duty to die that was predicated on the stigmatization of disability. Crane's "The Monster" (1898) disputes the assumption that the premature death of a disabled patient is natural. Wharton's *The Fruit of the Tree* (1907) critiques an act of "mercy killing" whose proponents instrumentalized the lives of disabled patients and populations. Lastly, Dalton Trumbo's *Johnny Got His Gun* (1939) pairs a war veteran's death wish with images of resurrected disabled patients, framing survival as both a personal and political challenge to a culture that associated disability with death. As I show in this chapter, as debates over euthanasia evolved over the early twentieth century, writers insisted on the fundamental value of disabled lives, gesturing toward how the medical professions might protect and help empower debilitated patients rather than causing them additional harm.

In focusing on health and social protest, I extend beyond the more individualized ways of understanding medicine that have animated some seminal strands of literature-and-medicine scholarship. For instance, Arthur Frank has shown how illness narratives can cultivate physicians' ethical understanding and moral sensibilities, while Rita Charon has demonstrated that literary scholars can enhance patient care by working to "singularize the care of patients, to recognize professionals' ethical and personal duties toward the sick, and to bring about healing relationships with patients, among practitioners, and with the public." Focusing on patients' perspectives, Ann Jurecic has emphasized the personal dimensions of illness, attentive to the ways that illness narratives foster empathy. While cultivating morals, ethics, and empathy have been a major focus of the medical humanities, scholars have also considered the epistemological skills that literature might help instill. For Sari Altschuler, a return to the porous boundary between literature and medicine in early America can help shift the medical humanities' focus from cultivating empathy to instilling more rigorous ways of knowing health.[22] In addition to discussions about the practical value of narrative for individual physicians, an emphasis on doctors' professional careers has been a central theme in criticism of nineteenth- and twentieth-century fiction, with a focus on how physicians' personal and professional aspirations and anxieties are negotiated.[23] While attentive to medical ethics, narrative, epistemology, and professionalism, in *Imagining Health* I consider how these issues all play out in fundamentally social contexts, demonstrating how authors foregrounded them to advance various versions of a collective politics of care.

As they encountered and portrayed professional medicine, American authors began to envision what a better system might entail, accomplish, and mean, yet doing so has never been straightforward. Their critiques are not always recuperable or simply to be celebrated. Some advanced sweeping visions of social change, while others offered more moderate, incremental reforms in the pursuit of a healthier nation. While many of their critiques resonate strongly today, they often struggled and sometimes even failed to transcend their own forms of hierarchical and exclusionary thinking. In what follows, I trace their trajectories—their successes, their compromises, and their failures—as they negotiated the boundaries between cultural expression and real-world medical advocacy, attempting to make a progressive politics of health more than a fiction.

CHAPTER ONE

The Cost of Care

RAYMOND CHANDLER'S SHORT STORY, from the 1950s, "It's All Right—He Only Died," illuminates the cruelties and contradictions within the US medical system. In this previously unpublished work, rediscovered in 2017, hospital clerk Iris observes a "transient"—a possibly intoxicated man struck by a truck. Strict regulations govern the private hospital where Iris is employed, including a requirement for a fifty-dollar deposit prior to admission. When a doctor arrives, he questions whether to allocate the hospital's resources and his own valuable time to this homeless case. Iris reminds him of the hospital's "millionaire donor," who stated at a board meeting, "The main thing to keep in mind is that this hospital is not run for charity." Recognizing that strict adherence to policy would secure his job—even at the expense of the patient's life—the doctor transfers the man to a county hospital, a public institution offering free services. However, by the time the patient arrives, it is too late; he dies in transit due to brain complications. "He might have been saved," remarks the receiving nurse to Iris the following day, "if they had operated on him immediately." The final twist reveals that the man had money concealed in his jacket that could have covered his treatment—if only Iris or the doctor had discovered it.[1] While the closure at the end of the story hinges on how he could in fact have paid for the treatment, ultimately the story contends that economic considerations should not obstruct access to care in the first place.

When *Strand Magazine* published this story in 2017, the *New York Times* positioned Chandler's bold critique as a prescient, scathing indictment of the post–World War II US healthcare system. The managing editor of Strand Magazine, Andrew F. Gulli, is quoted in the *Times* article arguing that "It's like Chandler is looking at the future and seeing how the health care crisis would get even worse. . . ."[2] At the same time, Chandler's story realistically portrays a crisis that was already unfolding within Chandler's historical moment. Furthermore, Chandler was not the first US fiction writer to produce this kind of critique, but he was contributing to an extensive and wide-ranging tradition of fiction that argues for expanded access to medicine, including, as this chapter focuses on, novels by Robert Herrick, Wallace Thurman, A. L. Furman, and Frank Slaughter.

While there is a long tradition of the provision of charitable medical care in the United States, in and around the early twentieth century, reformers and politicians attempted to introduce publicly funded medicine on a national scale. These efforts toward national health reform and particularly expanding health insurance have been characterized by incremental change amid resistance from both organized medicine and the general public. Although Theodore Roosevelt called for a national health coverage program as early as in the 1912 presidential election, the New Deal era ushered in a broader push for expanded access. At the National Health Conference organized by President Franklin Delano Roosevelt in Washington, DC (1938), a representative of the Steel Workers' Organizing Committee encapsulated the spirit behind these reform efforts in describing impoverished workers suffering from illnesses caused by conditions in factories, stockyards, and tenements. In an era of "industrial depression," she noted the prevalence of "dark, damp, ugly homes," "bad, inadequate food," and "little or no ability to pay for medical care." Paraphrasing the language of the Declaration of Independence, she asserted that medical care should be one of all citizens' "inalienable rights."[3] During the late 1930s and early 1940s, the Farm Security Administration developed medical programs—including health cooperatives and prepaid health plans in rural areas.[4] In the mid-1940s, President Harry Truman proposed a health reform agenda to ensure that all US citizens had health insurance, but his proposal was ultimately defeated. Throughout this period, even modest reform proposals were met with resistance from a medical establishment whose leadership largely sought to protect physicians' economic self-interest. In particular, these reform efforts encountered strong resistance from an increasingly organized business sector that included many medical professionals and the American Medical Association, which characterized the push for expanded coverage as a threat to US democracy by calling it "socialized medicine."

Authors have explored the cost of care as it has evolved through various stages of American capitalism. As early as the late nineteenth century, for example, the genteel Dr. May in Rebecca Harding Davis's "Life in the Iron Mills" (1861) is portrayed as having a limited perspective—shaped by the socioeconomic privileges of the medical profession—that prevents him from comprehending the reform efforts needed to alleviate the working classes' plight.[5] In Edward Bellamy's utopian novel, *Looking Backward: 2000–1887* (1888), doctors work for the state, so that "instead of collecting his fee for himself, the doctor collects it for the nation . . ."[6] In William Carlos Williams's "The Paid Nurse" (1939), a factory worker, after suffering an industrial accident, is denied the necessary care; instead of receiving proper treatment, he is ordered by the company nurse to return immediately to work. Outraged, the narrator–doctor exclaims, "What! . . . When he's in agony in the middle of the night from the pains of his burns, he has no right to get advice and relief? Is that what you mean?"[7] From representations of the effects of nineteenth-century industrialization on working-class health to the detrimental impacts of the early twentieth-century's harsh efficiencies on possibilities for compassionate medicine, a range of writers have pointed toward the problems emerging from a medical economy that privileges profit above care.

Novelists including Herrick, Thurman, Furman, and Slaughter are particularly remarkable for the extended socioeconomic critiques in their novels of medical care, focusing on how class inequality and the profit motive could corrupt professional medicine. The central issue at stake in their novels is what James Rorty stated in *American Medicine Mobilizes* (1939): "The simple fact is that whereas everybody needs a doctor, preferably before he is sick, the majority of our people today can't afford a doctor."[8] This "simple fact" opened up complicated and nuanced questions about access, affordability, and quality of care. In the work of these writers, plots of medical heroism are thwarted by political corruption and the monetization of health and life. While they portray individual experiences of illness and encounters with medical providers, they consistently situate the ethics of doctor–patient relationships within wider economic contexts. They challenge readers to consider not only how individual doctors exploited patients but also how unfettered capitalism and an underfunded public hospital system could undermine the mission of medicine. Critiquing a private medical system, they endorsed alternatives at both interpersonal and institutional scales.

The Gift of Health

Robert Herrick imagined healing as a gift, suggesting that medical care without payment from the patient might one day be integral to the US medical system. A realist novelist at the turn of the twentieth century, Herrick's fiction—while eschewing the muckraking tone of later realists—addressed pressing social issues. In novels such as *The Healer*, he examined the tensions and conflicts confronting a professional class of which he was a part, as a Harvard-trained professor of literature at the University of Chicago, within a rapidly industrializing economy. These professional dilemmas are dramatized through characters torn between realism and idealism, epitomized in *The Healer* by the clash between profit-driven medicine and efforts to provide benevolent care for the impoverished. The novel lends support to Philip Barrish's call for literary criticism to expand its focus beyond individual accounts of illness and care toward addressing medical systems. Toward that end, Barrish demonstrates how another of Herrick's novels, *The Web of Life* (1900) portrays a conflict between two competing visions of US medical care at the turn of the twentieth century: "a democratic profusion of health-care providers and options" versus a "health-care system that is centralized, rationalized, and directed from the top down by the so-called orthodox profession."[9] While Herrick examined competing capitalist models of professional medicine in *The Web of Life*, in *The Healer* Herrick challenged the very foundations of the capitalist medical system.

In *The Healer*, Herrick offers an extended meditation on healing as a selfless act of charity. The gift of care emerges at the novel's outset when Holden is summoned to perform surgery on Helen, a severely injured character. After saving her life, Holden marries her and leads her away from suburban life to the wilderness, where he establishes a rustic camp hospital by a mystical healing spring and administers care without expecting substantial repayment. Yet, this gift is continually threatened by commodification.

This commodification of medical care is depicted as a form of historical violence, including the appropriation of Indigenous peoples' lands for profit. When transporting Helen to the healing spring, Holden observes that sometimes "Indians" camp nearby, bringing their sick to the site: "They still have faith in the healing power of the Spring!"[10] Noticing "some withered tent poles," as well as "tin cans and yellowed newspaper," he infers that "white folks" have recently been in the area. According to Holden, the healing properties of the water have been stolen—the "modern world discovered them after its own fashion . . . even bottled the healing waters and sold them over the counter like everything else!"[11] This theft encapsulates the extractive nature of US consumer capitalism, as healing is exploited and packaged as a commodity.

Medical care has long been intertwined with the market economy, yet Herrick envisions care differently. Although hospitals in the late nineteenth and early twentieth centuries emerged as spaces of potential recovery—no longer merely last resorts for the impoverished or criminals—their benefits were not universally accessible, intensifying an awareness of increasing stratification in the medical care economy. By the early twentieth century, improved medical care was available but often only at prohibitively high costs. In this context, Herrick's depiction of the gift of care is best understood as a fantasy. Through the medium of literary fiction—and particularly within the romance genre—he imagines a model of non-market-driven care that, though possible, was becoming increasingly rare. The romance of healing is inaugurated at the healing spring, and Herrick acknowledges that it is perennially threatened within a consumer-capitalist economy.[12]

This tension is embodied in the conflict between Holden and Helen. Initially, Holden's gift of healing is intertwined with his love for her—it is his act of healing that sparks their romance—but eventually, Helen pressures him to profit from his gift, straining their relationship. For Helen, a gift is not meant to be "kept reserved"; she likens Holden's gift to "gold" that should be immediately mined, used, and exploited.[13] She argues that "when one loves ... one loves the whole world, too, a little."[14] Here, she specifically urges him to engage with the "world" of consumer capitalism in order to better provide for her. In contrast, Holden believes that entangling his gift with urban, profit-driven practices would destroy its integrity along with the very romance of healing.

These marketplace pressures begin to affect Holden's work—a narrative development through which Herrick links his character's experience to the increasing commercialization of medical care at the turn of the century. Initially, Holden resists the commodification of medicine, exclaiming, "doctoring—healing the sick—has become a trade!" and noting he saw this in medical school, with "big men using their reputation to bleed their patients who were rich enough to pay..."[15] Yet despite his reservations about profiting from his practice, he gradually earns more money as patients travel from the city to the healing spring. He expands the hospital's infrastructure by adding nurses, attendants, new buildings, and other elements of professional medicine. Through this trajectory, Herrick dismantles any illusions of doctors' transcendence above market forces. The hospital transforms into a kind of medical "machine in the garden," to borrow a term from Leo

Marx, as industry and capitalism encroach on pastoral space.[16] Although one critic described *The Healer* as having a "strong flavor of Thoreau,"[17] the pastoral ideal that Holden clings to through his representation of the healing spring ultimately becomes compromised by commercialization and industrialization; as he begins to sell his healing for profit, the mysterious power of his gift appears to be lost.

Some have argued that Herrick's emphasis on the gift economy reflects a desire to cling to a fading yeoman past amid an increasingly industrial and materialist culture,[18] yet his idealization of healing as a gift emerges not only from a general malaise with consumer-capitalist modernity but as a specific response to its effects on the working classes. When an impoverished patient named Eva consults Holden, she recounts how she was forced at a young age to endure "killing" factory labor in part because of her "invalid father"—much like "thousands and thousands of women" suffering the degradations of urban poverty.[19] Eva's testimony reveals the violent rupture produced by the transformation of healing from a gift into a commodity. After trying multiple doctors whose medicine fails to help her, she has now come to Holden. But realizing that Holden's services now come at a high price, she exclaims, "You cannot sell your gift. It will die if you sell that!"[20] She contrasts the care provided by Holden with the labor she has performed all her life: "I sold my labor . . . for my mother and sisters, but I did not sell a gift like yours!"[21] The commodification of care robs her of the healing that might have saved her, as gift-like forms of care become threatened by the ascendancy of industrial and consumer capitalism. Eva hopes healing would be protected from the profit motive, unlike her own labor, but this turns out not to be the case.

Ultimately, the harsh realities of the market economy overwhelm any possibility for a non-capitalist romance of medicine. When a forest fire destroys his wilderness hospital, Holden returns to the city and opens a practice. Blake Nevius has suggested that Herrick was perpetually torn between romance and realism, which were genres he regarded as distinct "moods."[22] Yet if he was conflicted himself, he also generated narrative tension—and conveyed his political message about modern medicine—through the friction he portrayed between these moods. As *The Healer* unfolds, the idealistic romance of the gift of care is eroded by market forces. The wilderness setting, Herrick's portrayal of Holden as the "Wild One," and his heroic rescue of Helen evoke an initial romantic ideal. But this ideal succumbs to the realistic pressures of commercial medical care as Holden's wilderness hospital becomes enmeshed in the marketplace. When he establishes a city practice, the urban medical marketplace is described as a "new wilderness" with its own "healing springs from laboratory to drug store."[23] Here, the reference to the wilderness no longer evokes pure romance, but connotes the unregulated, competitive nature of commercial medical care.

When Holden returns to the city, his gift of health is relegated to the realm of fantasy as he concedes to compromise. He acknowledges that the "broken Idealist" can only "dream of an unshattered Ideal."[24] Although this moment signals the foreclosure of political possibility, the idealistic vision of public medical care continues to propel the story forward. In the section of the novel taking place in the city, Holden envisions a new medical system, arguing that "the whole profession should be institutionalized—all medicine, all attempts at healing . . ." He contends that "the state should control the schools and the hospitals and regulate the numbers and the work of the doctors, and should establish everywhere public dispensaries as their headquarters . . . No doctor should be permitted to receive fees from his patients . . . Medical services should be free for all,—and compulsory—provided by society as a whole for its own preservation and betterment."[25] This radical proposal, anticipating later debates about medical coverage, reflects Herrick's desire to replace market-based care with state-controlled systems—which he views as the fullest expression of the gift of healing.

Other individually bestowed gifts are portrayed as well-intentioned yet ultimately inadequate within a profit-oriented medical system. For example, consider how in the city, Holden briefly works for a research institute devoted to studying nervous diseases among the working classes. Established by the wealthy philanthropist Mr. Elport with funds donated for the "aid of humanity," the institute leaves it to him to determine "the direction of the gift."[26] This charitable donation, described as a "gift" in a way that echoes Holden's care provided at the Healing Spring, represents an attempt to reform the urban medical economy. In contrast to his individual gift in the wilderness—which is largely an escape from capitalist pressures altogether—the professionalization of philanthropy is an attempt to redistribute resources. However, because it is only a minor gift, it risks assuaging liberal guilt while preserving the foundations of a consumer-capitalist medical system. Whereas Holden's gift of healing is based on a romantic, expansive vision of care, the research institute offers only a moderate, incremental change. Consequently, Holden concludes that such initiatives amount to little more than a "scratching of the surface" in addressing the problems wrought by market-driven medicine.[27] Disillusioned with the flawed economy of medical care, Herrick remains skeptical of the capacity for a donation to do much good. As one early reviewer noted, "there is an atmosphere of depression pervading the story that is hardly relieved by the opening of an 'institutionalized hospital,' where the doctors work for a fixed salary and the private fee is a thing of the past."[28] *The Healer* therefore concludes with a more complete vision of healing as a gift. Holden returns to the wilderness, accompanied by a young disciple whom he instructs in the art of the gift: "And I will teach you the great secret ... The will to give all! ... That is the secret."[29] In this final meditation, Herrick tips the narrative into the realm of a utopian fantasy: though the gift becomes increasingly vague, it also becomes increasingly expansive.

Critics immediately recognized the relevance of Herrick's critique of the medical economy. One British reviewer compared his approach in *The Healer* to Upton Sinclair's assault on American meat trusts in *The Jungle* (1905), noting that in *The Healer* Herrick "attacks the Medical Profession." In America," this reviewer noted, "the paid medical practitioner, according to Mr. Herrick, debases the high privileges of the profession: apparently he would have all medical men paid a fixed salary."[30] Responding to the particularly profit-driven nature of the American medical system, this reviewer was comforted by the sense in which the "evils he describes do not—we are glad to think—exist in England." Herrick's critique unsettled but also appealed to many in the medical community. A reviewer in the *Journal of the American Medical Association* claimed that Herrick viewed the medical system from a "socialist's viewpoint." Nevertheless, the reviewer noted "in spite of the fact that, the author gives expression to views that are not, altogether flattering to the medical profession, the novel is a fascinating one."[31] Dr. Lewellys Barker, a respected physician speculated to have inspired the character of Holden, conceded that while *The Healer* might seem socialist, Herrick "does not state these opinions as his own, merely placing the words in the mouth of his character." Barker advocated for a middle path in health reform—supporting increased coverage without the stigma of socialism—and pointed to emerging measures in Germany and England, such as an "invalid tax." He hoped that the changes articulated in *The Healer* would eventually come to fruition: "The time may come, as the morality and ideals of mankind reach high levels, when a physician, like other men, will be willing to do his best for the sake of doing it and not to gain primarily a monetary reward."[32] Although it remains uncertain how Holden's expansive "will to give all" will effect political change, Herrick implies—in a way that early medical reviewers recognized—that this kind of idealism would be essential for propelling the nation toward a more affordable medical system. The gift of care has to become systematized, even if the full realization of this goal appears as unlikely as fulfilling one's wildest dreams.

The Public Hospital and Private Practice

While in *The Healer* Herrick envisions publicly funded care as an idealistic, selfless gift, two decades later Wallace Thurman and A. L. Furman's *The Interne* offered a thinly fictionalized muckraking exposé that revealed the challenges faced by patients, nurses, and physicians within an underfunded public hospital system.

Thurman—a novelist, editor, playwright, and screenwriter of the Harlem Renaissance—experienced firsthand the deficiencies of an underfunded medical system. Sick as a child, stricken by the Spanish flu in 1918, he briefly studied as a pre-medical student at the University of Utah before succumbing to what he called a nervous breakdown.[33] Thurman died in the very City Hospital on Welfare Island that *The Interne* critiques. Experiencing what amounted to "incarceration," he wrote in a 1934 letter to Langston Hughes, "Being bedded among the proletariat is enough to make me or anybody become a rabid lover of the aristocrats." Thurman's point was not that care should be a luxury, but that the underpinnings of the medical system required fundamental changes. Despite improvements such as "more help and less dirt," in the modern hospital, he noted "it is still terrible" and he lamented that if these problems were "capital's fault," then "capital must be some villain."[34]

In *The Interne*, Thurman and Furman expose growing economic inequities in US hospitals. With the professionalization of medicine and nursing, increasing specialization, and urbanization, hospitals transformed from places where patients expected to die into institutions promising healing through advances like asepsis, anesthetics, laboratories, and X-rays. Yet modernization coincided with a shift from historically charitable care toward services for middle- and upper-class clients. Public hospitals, though still operating, faced severe financial challenges that rendered care for impoverished patients substandard. Public hospitals lagged behind their private counterparts—compromised by limited technology, organizational deficiencies, and corruption—a predicament dramatized in the portrayal of Memorial Hospital, a fictionalized version of City Hospital on Welfare Island (formerly Blackwell's Island). As hospital care became more advanced and costly, patients without sufficient funds could increasingly only expect to receive the right to free care from such public institutions, which led to immense financial pressure on them that could lead to institutional breakdown.[35] As the Great Depression deepened the strain on an already overtaxed system, public hospitals increasingly lacked the resources necessary to provide adequate care. In *The Interne*, the "intensification of an economic depression which gripped the entire nation" renders hospital facilities glaringly insufficient in terms of their ability to provide care for the sick.[36] In this context, *The Interne* portrays the various institutional failures within the public hospital that eventually lead the protagonist, a medical intern, to escape into private practice.

Some reviewers dismissed Thurman and Furman's realistic muckraking as overly sensational; one headline declared the work "Sensational But Ineffective Work: Aims to Expose Hospital 'Racket,' But Fails as a Novel,"[37] while another article argued that a "statistical account" might have offered a more effective critique.[38] Nevertheless, *The Interne* is significant for its portrayal of the real-world economy of medicine, particularly its impact on communities in poverty. As the intern protagonist Carl discovers, there is a fundamental difference between the care provided in the city hospital and that available to those who can pay—a class division that takes shape along lines of race, ethnicity, and religion, as Memorial Hospital's ambulance service serves "the more flagrant slum neighborhoods, grim complements to the progress of industry, in which were isolated the poorer Jews, Italians, Negroes, and Shanty Irish ... the other hospitals in the district were private institutions, catering only to patients who could pay."[39] Within this context, Thurman and Furman emphasize that the problems at Memorial Hospital stem from entrenched socioeconomic injustices rather than the failings of individual medical staff. The novel critiques the medical system as a whole—implicating institutional corruption and collective failure rather than individual negligence. In fact, most of the doctors and nurses are doing the best they can, which contributes to the novel's critique of medicine as an institution: the system is to blame, not individual medical actors. For this reason, despite all the corruption the novel points toward, the novel can still be dedicated to the "thousands of internes in public hospitals who conscientiously devote their lives and hearts to ease human suffering." Carl, recalling how his college professors had idealized the medical profession, criticizes them for having "glossed over the hardships, intimating these were the fault of individuals rather than a mass experience."[40] As medical negligence becomes rampant as a result of an overtaxed systems, the interns, despite their heroic efforts, become ensnared in corruption and institutional dysfunction. Over time, Carl himself becomes desensitized to the constant suffering with which he is faced: "Sprains, bruises, lacerations, childbirth, social diseases, contagious germ infections, even major operations . . . had become too commonplace for him to be emotional about."[41] Large-scale socioeconomic forces have desensitized Carl, limiting his own capacity for compassionate feeling.

Throughout, Thurman and Furman frame medical ethical issues as inseparable from economic ones. Though *The Interne* was initially criticized for being overly sensational, *The Interne* in fact positions seemingly sensational medical-ethical issues as ongoing, everyday problems within a subpar economy of care rather than aberrant exceptions to norms. For example, the novel details the issue of autopsy in economic terms. Memorial Hospital devotes its best resources to research on dead bodies. When a story circulates among the interns about a dying patient coerced into signing away his body for research, some interns justify this as a means to advance medicine—suggesting it might save "some other poor bastard from dying from the same thing"[42] Carl, however, is initially disturbed not only by the forceful coercion of patients, but specifically by the fact that better care is afforded to the bodies of the deceased than to those of living patients. This much is evidenced by the immaculate state of the morgue's refrigerators ("these refrigerators were the most clean, the most respectable, and the most modern equipment he had yet seen"), as opposed to the subpar conditions of the equipment in the rest of the hospital where the sick are treated.[43]

In addition to the issue of autopsy, the entanglements of medical-ethical issues with economic concerns become most evident in the novel's treatment of abortion. During the Depression, the abortion rate increased dramatically, as many couples increasingly felt they could not afford to have children.[44] Wealthier women, however, had higher abortion rates than working-class women because of abortion's high price.⁴⁵ As Karen Weingarten observes, twentieth-century novels often tie abortion to a shadow economy—depicting it as a transaction marked by "deception," theft, and exploitation,—while at the same time, reckoning with the high cost of abortions that made them inaccessible to many.⁴⁶ In line with this kind of critique, in *The Interne*, abortion is presented as being bound up in class politics. When Carl faces a fine for his involvement in selling prescription liquor to bootleggers, his fellow intern, Pete, suggests that he escape from the public hospital system altogether, and go to work for a wealthy abortion clinic. This would enable him to pay the fine and advance professionally. He could "retire, go to Europe, play around, study, then come back and be a swanky specialist." If not, he would "leave here broke and join the great multitude of penniless young physicians . . ."⁴⁷

Yet the socioeconomic questions at stake in Carl's decision are about more than Carl's career mobility. As Dr. Mason, a senior physician at the hospital, suggests, the ethics of abortion are entangled with wider economic questions. Mason does not express anti-abortion views, but he takes a position against performing abortions for the wealthy when not all women can afford them. Mason explains to Carl the potential implications of choosing to work for the wealthy clinic: ". . . where you're planning to go, you won't be helping the people who need that kind of help most. You'll be helping the idle rich."⁴⁸ If Carl goes to work for the wealthy abortion clinic, Mason suggests, he would be compromising on not only his morals but also his politics. Mason is attuned to the complexities of access issues within a capitalist economy of medical care. In this view, if Carl were to go to work for the wealthy abortion clinic, he would be contributing to a system that limits access for those most in need.

Ultimately, while not going to work for the abortion clinic for the wealthy, Carl opts for private practice as a means of self-protection. While the novel at first emphasizes how care has become impersonal, by the end of the novel, Carl's compassion is foregrounded but becomes separated from a sense of social responsibility and is instead only extended to his own family. After his love interest, the nurse Nora, becomes pregnant, she asks him to provide an abortion if he chooses the private route. Carl rejects this, viewing this prospect as tantamount to the "murder" of "his own child"⁴⁹ but still goes into private practice in a small town. The novel's resolution is both resigned and sentimental; images of privacy, domesticity, family, and reproductive futurism[50] lead to a disavowal of the need to reform the economy of medical care. Carl marries Nora, leaves the public hospital, and begins work as a physician for a manufacturing company's pediatric practice. This shift—from public care to private practice—reflects both personal burnout and a more fundamental exhaustion with a broken public medical system. Carl acknowledges that, like life itself, the practice of medicine is imperfect: "one could only do one's bit and hope that the little he could accomplish might minimize man's suffering."[51] Carl remains ambivalent about his choice, noting that one must "grit one's teeth" to cope with a life "devoid of meaning, fraught with ugliness."[52] In the final pages, as a new intern at Memorial Hospital learns to play bridge and drink liquor with his colleagues, the persistence of corruption is made clear—Memorial Hospital continues to function as a "machine" that prioritizes economic efficiency over care.

Toward the end of *The Interne*, Carl's epiphany is that "humanity was ill."[53] For a novel so concerned with the physical ailments of those denied quality care, this figurative portrayal of sickness—as a metaphor for universal suffering —captures the alignment between the corruption of the public hospital and a broader erosion of care. As Thurman and Furman show Carl's worldview contract to focus on self-protection, they express the anxieties that have rendered public medical systems so difficult to maintain. As they convey the general sense in which humanity itself can be understood as ill, the purview of compassionate care becomes much narrower, threatening to become limited to the individual family, the paying client, and the self.

National Health Insurance

While *The Interne* focuses on the subpar economic conditions of a specific hospital, Frank Slaughter's novel *That None Should Die* calls for more affordable access to medical care on a national scale, providing an extended encounter with the ideal of state-funded medicine that Herrick only mentioned in *The Healer*. Written in the wake of the 1930s social welfare debates—which saw several failed attempts to incorporate national health insurance into the New Deal's social security program—*That None Should Die* argues for expanded insurance, as the novel pairs an ethical commitment to charitable care for individual patients with a policy proposal for a national insurance program. In *That None Should Die*, Slaughter portrays the medical career of protagonist Dr. Ran Warren and his involvement in implementing a US health care plan that occupies a middle ground between capitalist and socialist systems. While Slaughter portrays the private medical economy as inherently flawed, he rejected a fully state-controlled system. Instead he imagined a solution that was partially private but still offered expanded, affordable coverage.

Drawing on his extensive medical background, Slaughter infused *That None Should Die* with firsthand knowledge of health care. Born in Washington, DC in 1908 and raised in North Carolina, he graduated from Duke University before attending Johns Hopkins Medical School, where he received his medical degree in 1930 at the age of 22. Later, he moved to Jacksonville, Florida. In 1934, as he started his surgical career in Jacksonville, Slaughter purchased his first typewriter. Shortly following this, he began writing best-selling novels.[54] Recognizing the need for a stable income, he resolved to remain in medicine until he could earn a living exclusively from writing. He later recalled, "I decided that if I ever got to the point where I could make a good living out of writing I would switch . . . But I didn't let up in my professional career."[55] Following the success of *That None Should Die*, he resigned from his post at Riverside Hospital in 1946 and became a full-time writer, while continuing to engage in public activities with the Florida Medical Association, and his local medical society, and lecturing to medical students when time permitted.[56] Even after leaving the medical profession, in 1946 Slaughter reportedly continued to read "everything new in medicine" and to research "medical developments constantly," which he felt contributed to the favorable reception of his work in medical journals. He prided himself on both his best-selling status and the factual accuracy of his novels, noting "it's accurate medicine; it's been researched right up to scratch."[57] Moreover, his deep knowledge of the political economy of medical care—gained while preparing for the American Board of Surgery's exams, during which he studied "extensively the then extremely controversial issues of hospital insurance and prepaid medical care"—informed his fiction, including *That None Should Die*.[58]

In *That None Should Die*, Slaughter presents medical care as an incredibly valuable resource in short supply. Before the Warren Plan is implemented, the private medical system forces the newly minted Dr. Ran Warren to confront the case of an impoverished child, Abie Bloomberg, from an immigrant Jewish family. Years earlier, Ran had promised Abie an operation for his leg injury, but because the overtaxed hospital where he works is constrained to admit "practically nothing but life-or-death cases."[59] Although Ran initially tries to turn Abie away, he eventually agrees to operate on him, ignoring the advice of a senior doctor and risking his job security all in an effort to challenge the profit-fueled structure of medical care. Slaughter dwells on Abie's surgery in minute detail, describing how Ran removes the "long piece of dead bone, the sequestrum," applies Vaseline to the wound, and sets a plaster cast to ensure that "healing would be rapid and complete..."[60] This fine-grained technical detail not only demonstrates Slaughter's mastery of medical material but also serves a thematic function by offering a brief reprieve from the bureaucracy, ethical dilemmas, and political struggles of changing the medical system. These scenes of healing, interspersed throughout the novel, function as self-contained narratives with tidy beginnings, middles, and endings, in stark contrast to the slow, unpredictable nature of medical reform—a process central to the novel's broader concerns. Despite the complexity of the political economy of care, medicine is presented as a crucial resource that demands better management.

This episode leads to a critique of not only Abie's treatment, but the way the high cost of care plays out more generally, as Abie's suffering comes to stand in for the effects of major flaws in US medicine. "Why should he have to go on being a cripple because his people couldn't pay for his treatment?" Ran demands, adding, "Here we are, the richest nation in the world, and people have to be lame or die because they don't have the money to pay doctors and hospitals."[61]

Throughout *That None Should Die*, Ran faces numerous additional challenges as he strives to protect patients' rights in a competitive, market-driven economy. For example, he encounters an ethical dilemma connected to the cost of care when one particular patient Mrs. McIntyre is referred to Dr. Sarnov, a physician known for performing dangerous Cesareans on women who do not require them. In the moment of *That None Should Die's* composition, Cesareans were increasingly prominent, as they were becoming particularly lucrative, even as insufficient attention was being paid to the risks involved.[62] Ran considers that exposing Sarnov's corrupt practices by informing her husband about these risks in order to save McIntyre would constitute a "direct violation of medical ethics." He is at first haunted by the oath he recited during his medical training ("that oath he had taken, the ancient oath of Hippocrates, what was its application here?"). But he then shifts his focus specifically to the "medical code," recalling that "one of the main provisions of that code was that the doctor should not speak ill of another before a patient."[63] He considers that he should not speak ill of Sarnov, even if it could mean saving McIntyre from harm. Eventually, however, these idealistic notions about professional codes designed to protect fellow doctors from competition with each other yield to the imperative of protecting at-risk patients. Initially, Ran privileges preserving the illusion of medical professionalism above fulfilling his ethical responsibility to McIntyre. When his wife, Anne, interjects with "medical ethics again?" Ran explains what he at first thinks is at stake: "There's no other profession where the members work together, helping each other, each minding his own business, as we do in medicine. What would happen if every doctor went around running down the rest of them to the patients? We'd soon degenerate into the worst of backbiting, cutthroat competition."[64] In time, however, Ran abandons this convoluted stance that prioritizes reducing competition among doctors over delivering proper, ethical care. The triggering incident occurs when Ran sees Sarnov claiming at a medical conference that none of his patients have died from his Cesareans, a claim Ran recognizes immediately to be false. At this point, he realizes that not just one life, but many are at risk from Sarnov's approach, which prompts Ran to speak out publicly against him. Ran's commitment to an aura of professionalism cultivated by respecting in public other physicians' authority cannot withstand his sense of social responsibility imposed by widespread illness and suffering.

While this moment reflects Ran's growing awareness of the derangements of profit-fueled medical care, *That None Should Die* also expresses a weariness of the alternative of completely government-controlled medicine. Slaughter was not immune from the pervasive anxieties about public medical care in the United States. While the first part of the novel privileges the notion of a right to medical care—expressed through scenes such as Ran's care for Abie and his exposure of Sarnov's corruption—the novel eventually morphs into the representation of a dystopian future of government bureaucracy in medicine that spirals out of control. Supporters of private medical care have championed patients' rights to choose their own doctors, a right the A.M.A. claimed was threatened by state-controlled medicine. More broadly, a liberal-individualist politics of negative rights—freedom *from* government interference—has been mobilized against government welfare measures, including compulsory health insurance, often casting "social rights" as part of socialism or communism.[65] *That None Should*

Die ultimately presents an argument for the right to care that is skeptical of excessive government intervention. Although Slaughter advocates for vulnerable patients, such as Abie, to have access to care, he suggests that a fully state-controlled system would obstruct rather than enable that right. His early critique of the medical system's setup makes his later embrace of even a partially private model all the more unexpected. Ultimately, Slaughter contends that when properly managed—with appropriate checks and balances on it—a hybrid economy of medical care, partially private and partially public, can be effective. In his portrayal of an imagined economy of state-controlled medicine, layers of bureaucracy come to dominate every aspect of licensing, practice, and policy, thereby obstructing the efficient distribution of care. Free, state-controlled medical care, in this vision, becomes a self-defeating fantasy, burdened by an overwhelming array of rules and regulations that thwart the noble work of healing. Notably, in *That None Should Die*, US citizens do not resist socialist medicine because of the redistribution of wealth via taxes but because they view the government itself as ineffective in managing medicine. In Slaughter's depiction, state-controlled medicine emerges as a "Frankenstein monster ... threatening to destroy the profession it was supposed to salvage."[66] Rather than being a monstrosity wrought by medical science, as in Mary Shelley's novel, it is government regulation that prevents medical care from being delivered effectively that becomes the monstrosity in question.[67]

To criticize completely state-regulated medicine—which Slaughter sees as an obstacle to good care—Slaughter returns to a scene of compassionate, sentimental care centered on a child.[68] Throughout *That None Should Die*, Slaughter deploys scenes of Ran's care for children to evoke the loftiest ideals of the profession. Ran's earlier care for Abie had highlighted the flaws of a faulty private system; later, within a state-controlled framework, Ran makes a house call to another child, Annie Hazlitt, who is struggling to breathe amid a diphtheria outbreak in her small town. At this point, Ran has failed to achieve a license that would permit him to perform specialized surgeries under a new overly regimented government system. However, he goes to Annie's home to save her with an operation anyway. The shift from hospital to domestic setting here is significant. As Ran approaches Annie's home and observes the burning lights of neighboring houses, he reflects, "each one of those lights might mean a sick child, complaining now of a sore throat or tossing in its sleep with fever."[69] Despite having lost his license to practice surgery under new government regulations, Ran defies the rules and operates on Annie. "What would you expect me to do?" he demands when accused of practicing without a license, "Stand by and see a child die from asphyxiation because of rules and red tape?"[70] In relaying Ran's argument, Slaughter anchors compassion for the vulnerable to a specific political stance: only a rogue doctor who challenges government overreach can deliver the care that suffering patients desperately need.

The notion that government-controlled medicine intrudes upon the sacred privacy of the doctor–patient relationship—especially jeopardizing the traditional setting of a house visit—has long been a focal point in arguments about the medical system. In 1948, for example, the AMA campaigned against President Truman's proposal for federal health insurance by enlisting public relations experts and featuring Luke Fildes' painting *The Doctor* (1891), which depicted a physician's house visit to a distressed child.[71] The accompanying caption, "Keep politics out of this picture," displaced questions of social and economic inequities by idealizing an increasingly obsolete scene of intimate care threatened by government interference.[72] Although Slaughter argues for expanded access to medical care through greater insurance coverage, he warns that too much government regulation in medicine could undermine the cherished aspects of individual, domestic care. "The day of the family doctor is gone," Slaughter would bemoan in 1972, predicting that "general practice as we know it will eventually disappear." In addition, he noted, that in *That None Should Die*, he had showed "that a government medical system would have all the faults that are inherent within an overly bureaucratic system ... Medicine is going through a rather political period.... I'm afraid a lot of the good aspects of individual medicine will be lost."[73] Slaughter's anxiety about bureaucratic intrusion compromising the doctor–patient relationship informs the scene of Ran's house call to Annie, underscoring the fear that medical care might become overly impersonal and mired in red tape as a result of too much government intervention.

Yet despite this anxiety, it is critical *That None Should Die* concludes with Slaughter reasserting the fundamentally political importance of an expanded social safety net within the medical system. While Slaughter ultimately rejects completely state-controlled medicine, he still insists on expanded access to medicine through increased taxes. Since socialist medical care has been demonized in the United States, Slaughter carefully distances his proposal from pure socialism, even as he argues for radically expanded access, and so he notes medicine would become "socialized" but only to a certain extent. Beginning to advocate for this "national system of health insurance," early in the novel, Ran tries to distinguish it from the specter of socialism while still promoting increased coverage. Ran envisions how, through a partial redistribution of resources—spearheaded by an alliance between the medical professions and political leaders—the best elements of private and public care can be combined. When critics label Ran's plan "pure socialism," he retorts that the medical economy is already partially socialized: "Who pays for the charity patients now? . . . Isn't it the city? Don't taxes support the hospitals and the free clinics? My plan would be a shift of financing; that's all. It would be a little more expensive, but the public would get a lot better treatment.[74]" He argues for extending forms of public funding in medicine already in place[75] to further tilt the balance toward increased access. In particular, he calls for medical practice to be "socialized to some degree for the benefit of the low-income patient."[76] While entirely socialist medicine proves to be dystopian, the solution of socializing medicine to a significant extent becomes reasonable, especially because it primarily extends tax-funded medical resources that are already in place within the US economy.

The trial implementation of the Warren Plan at the novel's conclusion embodies Ran's, and Slaughter's vision: a program that guarantees basic rights to care through minimal regulatory interference. The specific policy solution is predicated on a major redistribution of economic resources, explained in the novel's appendix, which breaks through the fictional narrative framing into a direct commentary on the real-world US economy of care. Under the Warren Plan, the medical care of low-income patients would be paid for by local or state governments—entailing "little more expenditure of tax money, since most of these people are already being cared for by charity hospitals in their areas"[77]—while insurance for middle-income patients would be "collected like a tax," leaving high-income groups to finance their own care.[78] Under this plan, lower-income patients are treated on par with those from higher-income groups.[79]

Throughout *That None Should Die*, Slaughter champions this liberal economic system and the reforms it would entail by asserting that it will protect the intrinsic value of medical care. He consistently emphasizes the good work doctors perform despite operating in a compromised system. In the final pages, the novel culminates in a poignant scene of surgery presented through Anne's dreamlike perspective. Having just regained her eyesight after a complication in childbirth—thanks, of course, to a medical operation—Anne envisions Ran and his colleagues pioneering the new system of medicine embodied in the Warren Plan. Slaughter writes, "as if her restored vision had acquired a more penetrating faculty, she could discern and interpret the faraway look in his eyes . . . She could see Ran in the operating theater again, gowned and masked, the blessed life-saving steel shining in his gloved hand. He was waiting for the anesthetist's nod, waiting to perform once more the miracle of surgery upon the figure beneath the sterile drawings. Working always toward the time when none should die for lack of the healing magic of the scalpel."[80] Here, Slaughter intertwines care and love, merging detailed medical descriptions with an imaginative, visionary tone that links the miraculous power of medicine to his specific policy proposal. Other authors of medical fiction with economic themes have been drawn toward intimate, ethical acts of care, including Holden's gift of healing in Herrick's *The Healer* and the kind of individual attention to patients that is jeopardized by institutional dysfunction in Thurman and Furman's *The Interne*. As is the case with these other novels, in *That None Should Die*, Slaughter interweaves attention to the ethics of compassionate, intimate care with large-scale questions of economic policy. Though he remains wary of excessive government intervention—expressed through depictions of red tape jeopardizing care—in the scene of Ran's care Anne, Slaughter envisions how intimate doctor–patient encounters may finally become aligned with progressive economic policies.

A minor bestseller, *That None Should Die* was well received by both the medical community and the public, as it would continue to be seen as prophetic regarding changes in the medical system as well as being perceptive about necessary reforms. While medical care was becoming more regimented, corporatized, and depersonalized with the consolidation of the medical-industrial complex later in the twentieth century,[81] *That None Should Die* would serve as a reminder that an investment in individual acts of compassionate, charitable care might extend into an attempt to remake the medical economy. Slaughter reflected on how the need for expanded public funding for medicine—as he had envisioned in *That None Should Die*—continued to resonate well beyond the novel's publication. In a 1967 issue of the *Journal of the American Medical Association*, Slaughter would compare the system of socialist medicine depicted in his novel to a future in which a failed proposal for health reform that was part of President Truman's Fair Deal program—the Wagner-Murray-Dingell bill—was passed. This piece of legislation, proposed by New York Senators Robert F. Wagner of New York, James E. Murray of Montana, and Representative John D. Dingell of Michigan in 1945 (after a similar proposal was made in 1943), would have enabled public medical care and hospitalization on a national scale, including compulsory health insurance for workers and their dependents.[82]

Alternatively, Slaughter considered the expanded access enabled by his fictional Warren Plan as the policy solution the nation needed. He presented the Warren Plan at the Conference on Ambulatory Care Services held by the Committee on Public Health of the New York Academy of Medicine in 1972 as a real-world solution to the current medical crisis. Slaughter noted that his fiction was initially dismissed as "medical heresy" with Bolshevist overtones.[83] He recalled that his "Warren Plan"—the proposal by Dr. Ran Warren for US medical reform—argued for a private rather than a fully state-controlled system, though it still incorporated regulation and public financing, and even this compromise initially raised concerns. While in *That None Should Die*, Slaughter had portrayed an idealistic young physician with a sense of social responsibility, Slaughter now observed that "it is a rather sad but . . . true commentary on a fundamentally idealistic calling that the social consciousness of most doctors is inversely related to their age and financial status."[84] Slaughter's plan, he noted, entailed "violating . . . the traditional shibboleths of free-choice-of-physician, fee-for-service, and individual solo practice. . . ."[85]

Over time, many doctors came to regard the Warren Plan as a reasonable policy solution. As Slaughter noted "even heresy may sometimes undergo metamorphosis into a gospel, as witness a 1971 Harris survey in which 55% of the people polled supported the principle of federal legislation to provide comprehensive health insurance, while a mail survey of doctors at the same time showed that 51% of the physicians agreed."[86] Slaughter justified the "economic feasibility" of his program, noting the resemblance of the Warren Plan to the rise of Health Maintenance Organizations (HMO), initially gaining popularity in the 1970s, as organized systems of medical care that would serve "an enrolled population for a fixed fee, agreed upon in advance": "Obviously," Slaughter noted, "these organizations bear a close resemblance to the Warren Plan, especially when you keep in mind that my plan was conceived at least 30 years, long before the present interest in HMO proposals came into being." Slaughter noted that recently health care costs had been "rising sharply," and he stood by his proposal for "medical care costs" for low-income groups to be covered by the government.[87] Slaughter continued to insist on the importance of increasing access to medical care, aligning his efforts with a growing movement for consumer choice, led by organized groups of consumer-citizens. He noted "were my plan being put into effect today, I would advocate joint control by physicians, hospitals, consumers and government at various levels."[88]

A report on Slaughter's conference contribution in the New York Academy of Medicine's bulletin indicated growing public support for a program akin to the Warren Plan. The New York doctor who wrote this report expressed his approval, noting that the "Warren Plan expressed in Slaughter's book *That None Should Die* would work now with appropriate modifications" as he valorized the "vision and the foresight embodied in statements Dr. Slaughter made in the late 1930s."[89]

Slaughter remarked in a 1973 radio interview that he was amazed to see that his Warren Plan that he had envisioned in *That None Should Die* could be adapted to his contemporary moment with only a few changes—encompassing group medicine and national health insurance.[90] Slaughter still expressed his concern with "socialized medicine" noting that *That None Should Die* contained a "large section on a theoretical or futuristic socialized medicine setup" intended to expose the "evils of bureaucracy." Nevertheless, he emphasized that the medical system has been 'grossly inefficient . . . We spend something like eighty-eight billion dollars a year for something like all phases of medical care" and "we should be able to give the people of the United States . . . the best health record in the world." Despite spending a great deal on medical care, he noted, the US lagged behind many nations in health outcomes, even countries that spent much less on medical care. True to the vision he had expressed in the Warren Plan, Slaughter remained as weary of excessive government regulations as he was of a fully private medical system that left too many citizens without reliable care.

As the cost of care became an increasingly visible policy issue in the US as a result of advances in medical science that were not available to all, writers such as Herrick, Thurman and Furman, and Slaughter demonstrated the transformative potential of professional medical work beyond the rigid constraints of an exclusively private medical system. While Herrick, and Thurman and Furman showed how individual characters navigated between systems of profit-fueled and charitable care , Slaughter imagined American society as a whole transitioning between private care, socialist medicine, and a hybrid, private/public system. These authors all illustrated how private health care has been but one option among many and, through varying strategies, called for significantly expanded access to medicine. To do so, they privileged compassionate care, but at a social rather than only an individual level. That is to say, an emphasis on the gift of healing, charity, and sentimentality had to extend beyond singular acts of care between doctors and patients and encompass institutional efforts toward implementing publicly funded medicine.

CHAPTER TWO

Professional Medicine and Racial Protest

HARLEM RENAISSANCE WRITER MARITA Bonner's short story "Drab Rambles" (1927) conveys a powerful critique of prejudice in the medical system, opening with a series of urgent declarations: "I am hurt. There is blood on me. You do not care. You do not know me. You do not care. There is blood on me. Sometimes it gets on you. You do not care. I am hurt. Sometimes it gets on your hands—on your soul even. You do not care. You do not know me. You do not know me, you say, because we are different. We are different, you say. You are white, you say, and I am black..."[1] In the narrative that follows, Bonner depicts Jackson—a patient nearly denied treatment at a public clinic by a white doctor—suffering from an abnormally rapid heartbeat. The doctor eventually offers to try to help, but the inadequacy of his care becomes positioned as a form of violence; his failure to recognize the extent of Jackson's suffering figuratively leaves blood on his hands. Bonner situates this scene of medical neglect and harm within the context of the broader social forces that affect African Americans' health, insisting that such problems cannot be resolved through partial measures or wholly individualized resolutions. When the doctor advises Jackson to seek a job other than digging ditches to protect his heart, Jackson retorts, "I had to dig ditches because I am an ignorant black man. If I was an ignorant white man, I could get easier jobs. I could even have worked in this hospital."[2] In addition to subtly arguing here for the need for increased representation of Black doctors within the profession, the story calls attention to a white-dominated medical profession's complicity in harmful and slowly lethal forms of neglect. Within this context, Jackson's act of lighting a pipe at the end of the story—despite the doctor's warning not to do so in order to protect his health—and his misplacement of the doctor's prescription that, he had noted, might "help some," underscore the inadequate nature of the care the doctor has offered.³ The ending of the story charts a vision of rebellion against medical injustices that cannot be addressed by individuals changing their behaviors alone, but instead require institutional and social resolutions.

Numerous other early- to mid-twentieth-century authors confronted and critiqued a white-dominated and largely segregated medical establishment, and, similarly transcending an emphasis on self-care, they elaborated on the potential of alternative versions of professional medical care anchored to racial justice. Writers including Charles Waddell Chesnutt, Walter White, and Ralph Ellison not only critiqued a deeply flawed medical system, but they also examined how revised forms of professional medicine could contribute to liberation. They extended earlier critiques of racist science and medicine while adapting to an era of medicine's rapid professionalization,⁴ centering modern, professional medicine in their fiction, and rather than eliding or opposing conventional medical authority entirely, rendering reclaimed forms of it as mechanisms to transform the politics of health.

Just as Bonner's "Drab Rambles" briefly calls attention to the obstacles that African Americans faced in entering the medical profession, with Jackson's comment about not being able to work in a hospital job, these writers insisted on the importance of African American representation within the medical professions at a time in which such representation was both newly visible and yet constantly imperiled. While African American physicians had long played a role in the medical field, it was not until after the Civil War that Black medical colleges were established. Beginning in the late 1860s, and into the twentieth century, a politically engaged, professional class of African American physicians emerged prominently.⁵ Yet, their participation in the medical field was made vulnerable by the profession itself, whose leadership marginalized non-white care providers and devalued Black medical education. A report in 1910, written by Abraham Flexner under the auspices of the Carnegie Foundation, encapsulated this process of marginalization, striking a major blow to progress. Intended to produce higher admissions and graduation standards in medical education, and to centralize medical institutions, the Flexner report also left open only two African American medical schools, and proposed that the practice of Black physicians should be "limited" by their "own race."⁶ While Black physicians continued to enter the field, they were met with professional obstacles and widespread resistance. Chesnutt, White, and Ellison, taking up medical themes, and attuned to these developments, brought African American physicians into literary representation while conveying a sense of the conflict-ridden professional cultures in which they had to operate.

In addition to emphasizing the importance of increased representation at a critical juncture in the evolution of modern medicine, they paid attention to broad social and political forces influencing Black patients' and populations' health, including segregation and continuing acts of medical violence, that, as relayed in Bonner's story, left American medicine itself with blood on its hands. These writers paid attention to the relationship between modern medicine and debates about whether educated Black professionals could or would aid the masses, efforts to expose the illegitimacy of the "separate but equal" doctrine, and ways to account for and mitigate against the impacts of infrastructural and environmental injustices on Black communities' health. Increasing professional medical representation was critical, then, but as part of a broader effort to eradicate the prejudiced underpinnings of the medical field.

Professionalism and Prejudice

In 1914, Charles Chesnutt—who had by then become established as a seminal novelist—delivered a speech entitled "The Ideal Nurse"[7] at a Chicago YMCA to the graduating class of the Provident Hospital training school for nurses. Established in 1891 with the explicit aim of combating racism in medicine, the school provided a platform for Chesnutt to assert that work in nursing was about more than earning a living; it could also be an ethical and humanitarian vocation. The movement taking shape in the early twentieth century for Black-led hospitals can be seen not solely as a symptom of segregation but also as part of a broader tradition of collective empowerment.[8] While Chesnutt acknowledged that many nurses might be driven by "economic necessity—the need to earn a living," he contended that an equally important motivation was the "wish to do something for humanity."[9] Citing Florence Nightingale as an exemplar—who, by supporting the British Red Cross, devoted her life to improving the lives of the sick and suffering—Chesnutt argued that the humanitarian potential of nursing emerges not only during national crises, such the Civil War, but also in moments of routine, compassionate care provided by nurses in homes and hospitals. He observed that the modern hospital served as a haven where the "sick and wounded poor," criminals, and victims of crime could find "rest and recuperation."[10] Beyond acquiring technical knowledge in physiology, anatomy, anesthetics, and antisepsis, nurses were expected to cultivate charity, sympathy, and devotion. According to Chesnutt, the nurse–patient relationship was central to the medical professions' collective impact: "after all," he noted, "society is composed of individuals, and the more individuals are nursed back from illness or injury to health and soundness, the better will be the general tone of the community . . ."[11]

Chesnutt's speech, however, did not simply offer a universalizing endorsement of these nurses' work and their impact on American society in general. He specifically addressed race relations, embedding his discussion of nursing ethics within the broader struggle for a just, desegregated medical system. He urged the nurses to recognize that they were engaging in "the great work of humanity, the great work of social uplift."[12] Yet he warned them that "because of your race, or rather because of the mean and unworthy prejudice against your color, the field of employment in most hospitals will be closed to you."[13] He further noted that the one would think that in the "Southern United States, where white people are accustomed to having colored people wait upon them," Black nurses "would be in demand" remarking that it would seem "a refinement of race prejudice for a family which would employ a colored cook or butler or maid, to object to the presence in the household of a colored nurse."[14] But he observed that many Black professional nurses' services were denied by white families. He also noted that the work of a "trained nurse represents a higher type of service" than the work of butlers or maids, and for this reason professional nurses such as those whom he was addressing could be seen as threatening to white people. As for doctors, who are even higher in the professional hierarchy, they faced even more barriers in employment.

For these reasons, Chesnutt suggested that it could take exceptional, life-or-death scenarios for Black nurses' services to be enlisted by prejudiced white families. He noted that recently, a South Carolina statesman had introduced a bill to "prohibit colored nurses from attending white patients."[15] A newspaper report accompanying this bill described how a white child's family initially refused care for the child by a Black nurse but requested her services as a last resort in the face of the child's life-threatening illness. Chesnutt argued that such an act of care served not only society in general but specifically the Black community.[16] As he noted, this nurse "was able not only to perform a service for humanity, but in a larger sense, to render a valuable service to her race" by lifting "the race that much higher on the economic and social scale."[17] For Chesnutt, professional work in nursing was crucial not only as a mode of acquiring individual status and class mobility but also as a strategic mechanism of racial advancement. While saving a white child from the "jaws of death," for Chesnutt the nurse's life-saving care was not only valuable because an innocent life was saved but because of the way that in saving the child, this nurse advanced her own community.[18]

Chesnutt suggested that the nurses whom he was addressing would ideally attend to the social welfare of patients who would otherwise lack access to medical care, including those neglected in increasingly congested cities, and particularly, impoverished Black communities.[19] Despite the professional obstacles faced by nurses and barriers to access to medical care faced by patients, Chesnutt noted that according to an issue of *Negro Year Book* in 1913, there were in the United States "sixty-three hospitals" conducted both "for" and "mostly by" African Americans, "which must give employment to several hundred nurses."[20] Toward the end of his address, he challenged the Provident Hospital training school nurses to demonstrate their capacity for their profession in the following terms: "Think of your great grandmother, who when she had a pain in the stomach thought she was conjured; who could not earn in a month as much as you earn in a week; and probably did not get what she earned."[21] In doing so, Chesnutt anchored his idealized vision of professional care to the process of overcoming racial injustices affecting earlier generations' health. A history of uncompensated labor leading to suffering and sickness seemed to be giving way to possibilities for compensated professional work that could now be oriented toward communal empowerment and health.

In fact, Chesnutt recounted how a trained nurse was critical to his own recovery from illness. In June 1910, Chesnutt had suffered a "slight stroke" and was hospitalized for it.[22] After that, this illness kept him confined to his bed for a month.[23] "I shall always remember with pleasure," he recounted in his speech, "the soft-voiced, gentle-handed little nurse who washed me and dressed and fed me and read to me as though I were a child for several weeks of such a convalescence following several other weeks in a hospital."[24] Here, Chesnutt centered himself receiving the sympathetic attention of a nurse, comparing his dependency on a nurse to his assumption of a child-like state in a way that would have implicitly begged his listeners to consider the relationship between the care he received and the care requested, only as a last resort, for the child in South Carolina. Through this framing, Chesnutt privileged acts of care by and for members of Black communities as a critical supplement to attempts at gaining professional recognition from white patients and families when such attempts were met with overwhelming resistance.

In *The Marrow of Tradition* (1901), Chesnutt had begun to articulate the themes that he later addressed in "The Ideal Nurse," gesturing toward the ways that acts of medical care could empower communities despite major obstacles. In *Marrow*, Chesnutt depicts physician William Miller, who, after completing his medical education in Paris and Vienna, returns to the fictional town of Wellington to establish a hospital. William's wife, Janet, is the biracial half-sister of Southern aristocrat Olivia Carteret. Her husband, Major Carteret, a newspaper owner with white supremacist leanings, vies for political power. Meanwhile, Josh Green—traumatized by the murder of his father by the white supremacist George McBane—seeks revenge and is treated for an injury at William's hospital. As Carteret and his associates incite a riot that leads to William's hospital being burned down, Josh is killed, though only after he fatally wounds McBane, who has attacked him, in self-defense. The novel concludes with William preparing to operate on Dodie, the child of the Carterets—a scene that is shadowed hauntingly by the recent loss of William's own son to the white supremacist mob.

Criticism of *Marrow* has often focused on Chesnutt's perceived conservatism and gradualism. William advocates, to an extent, for gradual change—in contrast to Josh Green's commitment to combative resistance. Stephanie Browner argues that, for Chesnutt, William symbolizes racial uplift and benefits from a form of class privilege that distances him from his injured, working-class patient.[25] Susan Danielson asserts that although professionalism "promised . . . a neutral, scientific ground from which to begin the process of social amelioration, based not on traditional prejudices but on reasonable community needs for service," William's optimism about assimilation is ultimately "rebuffed by the northern physician's acquiescence to white southern tradition." In a segregated society, Danielson suggests, William's emphasis on professional assimilation is bound to fail. When a riot erupts at the novel's end—threatening and ultimately destroying William's hospital—his "professional commitment to racial uplift" is exposed as "individualistic," "self-serving" and "shallow."[26] Noticing a similar anxiety about professionalism, Brian Sweeney contends that in *Marrow* Chesnutt "tentatively endorses the professionalist sentiments of many elite African Americans . . . while at the same time expressing doubts as to the power of professionalism's ideals of meritocracy and public service to realize a more racially egalitarian bourgeois social order."[27] Whether or not critics view Chesnutt as endorsing William's sense of his medical professionalism, their readings share a sense of the perceived failure of that professional sensibility to address the root causes of racial prejudice. As the doctor who, amid white supremacist rioting, instructs his community to "give it up, boys, and wait,"[28] it is not wholly surprising that critics have characterized William's orientation toward professionalized uplift as moderate and conservative. In the late nineteenth and early twentieth centuries, uplift ideology was articulated through the insistence on assimilation, "respectability," and self-help by upper- and middle-class African Americans. As Kevin Gaines has shown, post–Reconstruction uplift involved elites claiming "status, moral authority, and recognition of their humanity by distinguishing themselves, as bourgeois agents of civilization, from the presumably undeveloped Black majority."[29] Stephen Knadler observes that attempts at what he calls "medicalized uplift"—including moralizing hygienic reform and the encouragement of the regulation of health and sanitation—find expression in novels such as Chesnutt's *Marrow*.[30]

At the same time, if Chesnutt registers a politics of medical uplift in *Marrow*, he also transcends the elitist trappings of this kind of discourse, explicitly focusing on the threats to Black communities' health posed by white supremacist violence. For Chesnutt, professional doctors direct their efforts not only toward securing their own economic mobility but also toward combating white supremacism and racial violence. As Andreá N. Williams notes in *Marrow*, "black Americans are subject to white violence regardless of their class status" because "white supremacy is embedded in the marrow of tradition."[31] This focus on the overriding influence of white supremacy is especially evident in the novel's representation of medicine. As William's hospital—where he treats the impoverished patient Josh Green—is burned down by a white mob following repeated attacks on his practice, Chesnutt demonstrates that Black health, across class lines, is undermined by white violence. In response, while *Marrow* may reflect elements of medical uplift and elitism, Chesnutt also articulates a radical form of racial protest through his critique of medical segregation and his vision for the transformative potential of William's hospital.

Ultimately, Chesnutt endorses those aspects of William's professionalism that unfold as powerful forms of resistance against white supremacism, and there are some key moments in which the very definition of medical professionalism is explicitly at stake that reveal this. When William is at first called to care for Dodie, the scene anticipates Chesnutt's comments, years later, in his speech to the graduating nurses of Provident Hospital's training school, about a particular nurse's life-saving care for a white child being called for—but only as a last resort. In this scene in *Marrow*, a physician named Alvin Burns tries to convince his colleague Price to allow William to operate on Dodie. From the outset, Burns thinks, "If William were going as a servant, to hold a basin or a sponge, there would be no difficulty; but as a surgeon—well he wouldn't borrow trouble."[32] When he is met with expected resistance from Price, Burns says he invited William in a "strictly professional capacity, with which his color is not at all concerned."[33] He reiterates that his "professional honor is involved" and that this is a matter of "principle, which ought not to give way to a mere prejudice." But Price denies William's services. Burns insists that "professional honor is involved . . . It is a matter of principle, which ought not to give way to a mere prejudice."[34] As William is not allowed to provide professional care prejudice does indeed win out in this scene over professionalism. But in his very suggestion that professionalism is "not at all concerned" with "color," Burns' articulation of his liberal, color-blind ideology betrays that he himself does not understand the meaning of professionalism to William. For William—and for Chesnutt—medical professionalism could be about more than assimilating and gaining recognition from white physicians. In fact, William sees his professional duties as serving the communities injured by precisely the kind of violence Carteret is complicit in. Rather than supporting a version of professionalist ideology that obscures issues of racism and resistance, William's sense of professionalism takes shape through his emphasis on the provision of care for communities who have been injured by racial violence. The concept of medical professionalism is not at fault; rather, William's white colleagues' avowedly professional sensibilities are corrupted by white supremacist ideologies.

A version of William's professional healing as a subtle form of racial protest emerges at the foreground of the novel in his treatment of Josh

Green at his hospital, where the two forge a powerful political allegiance. When Josh arrives with a wounded arm from a fight with a sailor, the sailor is promptly taken for medical care while Josh is left in pain. Earlier, the KKK attacked his family, and William notes the traumatic effects of this violence: "the old wound still bleeding, the fruit of one tragedy, the seed of another."[35] In the context of this injurious history, William must serve both as a doctor and a political leader; in fact, the two aspects of his practice become inextricably linked.

In the conversation that unfolds, William balances compassion and nonviolence with an approach that privileges healing as a means of self-defense and power. In fact, his combination of restrained professionalism and emboldened protest resonates with Josh's attitude. Although Josh recounts striking back at the sailor who attacked him, he ultimately refrains from killing him—recognizing that his assailant might have dependents and therefore compassionately sparing his life. In the hospital, when Josh describes earlier injuries inflicted on him and his family by McBane's men and pushes for the need to fight back, William dismissively diagnoses him as "feverish" while laying a "cool hand" on his brow and advising against further violence.[36] Later, when the white supremacist riot erupts, William similarly characterizes that violence as a kind of "fever," advising, "It is a fever; it will wear off to-morrow, or to-night. They'll not burn the schoolhouses, nor the hospital—they are not such fools, for they benefit the community . . ."[37] By framing both Josh's resistance and the mob's proclivity toward violence as transient eruptions within a society committed to the public good, William implies that the anger that spurs both is socially disruptive and must be carefully "cooled" down. William's moderation is not a sign of weakness but a deliberate strategy for self-protection and survival. Moreover, William does not entirely reject the use of physical force against white supremacist violence; he acknowledges that the healing he provides may even enable such force. William admires Josh's desire for revenge, observing that Josh "could remember an injury" and "shape his life to a definite purpose, if not a high or holy one."[38] Furthermore, he questions the limitations inherent in his own moderate stance when he notes that Josh "was willing to give up his life to a cause. Would he be equally willing . . . to die for it?" When William tells Josh to "keep quiet" until his arm is healed, warning that otherwise he "may never be able to hit any one with it again,"[39] his remark seems to be made in jest, and yet, later, when the mob attacks the hospital, Josh indeed strikes rioter McBane with his "powerful right arm."⁴⁰ This essential detail explicitly links healing with self-defense, as Chesnutt evokes the earlier scene through the reference to the arm, aligning professional healing with physical resistance.⁴¹ Although treating a patient is, in one sense, simply a doctor's professional duty, Chesnutt adds a political dimension to this act of healing through the image of the arm that strikes back.

While William's healing is itself an act of resistance, it is persistently challenged by the cruelties of segregated medical care. In fact, the depiction of Josh's right arm is not the sole reference to a "right arm" in the novel; Chesnutt describes a white character's injured right arm as well. Initially, as Carteret frantically searches for a doctor during the riot to save Dodie, a newly graduated medical student informs him that a more senior, white doctor, Yates, is unavailable because, amid the chaos, his frightened horse threw him from his buggy, breaking his right arm.⁴² Chesnutt compels us to view Yates's' broken arm—which delays Dodie's care—in light of the parallel injury sustained by Josh, which nearly goes untreated.

Amid these conditions, the connection points between medical professionalism and social protest foregrounded in the scene of William's healing of Josh continue to surface elsewhere in the novel. When William encounters a victim of the white supremacist riot that attacks his community, his professional impulse to help—despite being outside the hospital setting—is vividly recalled: "every professional instinct urged him to stop and offer aid to the sufferer . . ."⁴³ Yet, driven by the need to protect his family, he leaves the wounded man untreated. Soon after, though, he finds Jane—the nursemaid of the Carterets who provides care for Dodie throughout the novel—dying on the sidewalk. Chesnutt writes that "his heart came up in his mouth. A second glance revealed that it could not be his wife. It was a fearful portent, however, of what her fate might be. The war had reached the women and children."⁴⁴ Here, William's professional mission to heal the Black community converges with the same kind of sentimental care that initially led him to rush back to his family. But William cannot fully heal the injuries inflicted upon his community, and so he remains "sick at heart."⁴⁵

While privileging William's efforts, Chesnutt also expresses skepticism that African Americans' entry into the medical profession will automatically earn them respect from white physicians or patients. From the outset, white supremacist ideology in *Marrow* undermines collective health by distorting the meaning of medical professionalism. Although William's professionalism serves as a mechanism of empowerment for his community, white supremacist ideologies distort the sense of what it entails. In *Marrow*, William confronts numerous obstacles to his professional reputation due to discrimination. Initially, he believes that if allowed to operate on more patients, his status might be recognized: William, Chesnutt writes, "liked to believe that the race antagonism which hampered his progress and that of his people was a mere temporary thing . . . and that when a colored man should demonstrate to the community in which he lived that he possessed character and power, that community would find a way to enlist his services for the public good."[46] Yet the novel registers caution about this assessment, as white patients largely refuse his services: "except in the case of some poor unfortunate whose pride had been lost in poverty or sin, no white patient had ever called him for treatment."[47] In Wellington, "white physicians were not unwilling to share this unprofitable practice" with a Black doctor only if deemed "worthy of confidence."[48] The qualified language in these instances registers professional acceptance that is only partial, and often only offered as a last resort.

Medical professionalism promised a route toward class mobility, but as Chesnutt relays, the emergence of a professional identity was constantly met with suspicion and resistance—even as less professionalized forms of care were readily accepted. This point comes into focus when he describes a nurse aboard a car reserved for white passengers, whom William encounters on his way to Wellington. Since he is threatened with having to move to a different car, when he sees her, William ponders how white people "do not object to the negro as a servant. As the traditional negro,—the servant,—he is welcomed; as an equal, he is repudiated." Here, Chesnutt contrasts the way that professional care is rejected by white people while non-professional, or less formally professionalized, care is often readily made recourse to. Whereas professional care is seen to threaten the white professional class status and is therefore only turned to infrequently, non-professional care is constantly taken advantage of.

William's provision of care for Dodie might seem to promise professional recognition, but finally the implication is that William's professional services are being exploited. When William is asked to operate on Dodie, he interprets the request as evidence that "having recognized his skill, the white people were now ready to take advantage of it."[49] The phrase "take advantage" is ambiguous—suggesting either recognition or exploitation—but Chesnutt prods us toward the latter interpretation. When Carteret summons William to care for Dodie, Chesnutt conveys his thought process: "that this doctor was a man of some education, he knew; and he had been told that he was a man of fine feeling—for a Negro—and might easily have taken to heart the day's events. Nevertheless, he could hardly refuse a professional call—professional ethics would require him to respond."[50] Like Burns, Carteret fails to grasp that for William, professionalism is characterized not by neutrality or a desire for assimilation but by his commitment to racial justice. More specifically, as seen in his care for Jane, William's professionalism is intertwined with his capacity for deep sentimental feeling—a quality Carteret minimizes when he claims that William may be a man of feeling, but that that capacity for feeling for his community would not interfere with his professionalism. In his "heart"—as readers witness through his compassionate care for Josh Green and later his sympathetic care for Jane, which makes his "heart" come up "in his mouth" before her death and then leaves him "sick at heart" after it—William aspires to heal his community; it is this commitment to sentimental care that in fact constitutes his professional ethics. Whereas Cartaret sees care for Dodie as an expression of professional ethics, William's ethical allegiances are largely directed elsewhere. His professional identity, influenced by a sentimental form of racial protest, is directly challenged when Carteret, only acting as a last resort, seeks his aid. This prompts William to exclaim, "You have tried all the others—and then you come to me!" At this moment, Carteret laments that he did not expect "professional jealousy" to hinder care for his son, insisting that he sought William's "professional services" for his only child. Yet it is not "professional jealousy" that makes William reluctant to save Dodie; rather, William is anxious that his professionalism is being abused while life-threatening violence against the Black community—including the murder of his own child that haunts the scene of care for Dodie—remains unchecked.

In pointing to the limited professional acceptance received by William, *Marrow* anticipates the remarks Chesnutt would later make in "The Ideal Nurse" about the cruelty of families who readily would accept the services of Black maids or servants yet refused those of professional Black nurses. In *Marrow*, even when African American medical professionals are called upon, acts of care may replicate the historical exploitation of less professionalized care work when racist harms go unaddressed. As with Jane's care for Dodie, William is expected to show compassion for the Carteret family's vulnerabilities even as his community is under assault by those same families. William's care for Dodie also mirrors the scene of another young nurse trained at his hospital, who provides care for Dodie and regards her work as "purely a matter of business" though she is underpaid ("they gave her nothing but her wages, and small wages at that"). Ultimately, William, like Jane and the trained nurse, provides care for a white family while being treated in a way that precludes a complete recognition of his expertise. Consequently, in terms of the nurse he encounters on the train—who is permitted to ride in the car reserved for white passengers—the implication is that he is in a more similar position with her than he initially thought to be the case. When William is ultimately called upon to save Dodie's life out of compassion and professional decorum, his professionalism is being exploited. The point is not that care should be withheld from an innocent patient such as Dodie, but that alongside such individual acts of compassion, medical segregation and racial violence must also be addressed. The recourse to William's professional medical care may create a caveat within a segregated system, serving white care-related needs, but without challenging segregation's fundamental basis. Ultimately, even in the practice of professional medicine, William's care for Dodie risks replicating the exploitation of manifestations of less formalized and professionalized care work that Chesnutt critiques.

The ending of *Marrow* is haunting not because it leaves the plot unresolved, concluding as it does before we learn the outcome of William's operation on Dodie and therefore whether he will live or die, but because the ending diverts attention away from the ongoing social issues that the novel has portrayed. The medical care provided for Dodie cannot address the problems of segregation, exploited care, and racial prejudice in medicine that Chesnutt has conveyed. The scene of William's care for Dodie prefigures Chesnutt's later remarks in "The Ideal Nurse" regarding the fraught politics of cross-racial acts of care in the South. With this in mind, it is critical to recall that William's earlier healing of Josh anticipates the guidance Chesnutt would also offer in that speech about acts of care within the Black community as sources of collective empowerment. In fact, the novel's privileging of care by and for the Black community also anticipates Chesnutt's later commentary on his own state of vulnerability and the care that he received from a professional nurse when he fell ill, reducing him to a child-like state.

Chesnutt's own valuation of this care is explicitly connected to a mission that privileged racial justice—as opposed to the scene of care provided for the child, Dodie, whose family inflicts violence while expecting compassion in return. Throughout *Marrow* and Chesnutt's implicit reflections upon it in "The Ideal Nurse," Chesnutt conveyed possibilities for a politics of care that he hoped would transcend the constraints of uplift, assimilation, and unreciprocated compassion, a form of care that would unfold instead as collective resistance against injurious hatred.

Desegregating Medicine

By the early twentieth century, medical segregation was firmly entrenched, and Walter White, the novelist and civil rights activist who served as the Executive Secretary of the National Association for the Advancement of Colored People (NAACP) from 1929 to 1955, addressed it in his literature and his reform efforts. As did Chesnutt, White focused on the impossibility of individualized and often melodramatic resolutions to social problems. Instead, he explicitly demanded fundamental changes to the medical system predicated on both amplifying diversity in professional representation and implementing national reforms to the medical system.

The violent, lethal effects of a segregated medical system were deeply personal to White. In an unpublished essay recounting his father's death after a car accident, White described how, while unconscious, his father was taken to a "modern, well-equipped 'white'" hospital in Atlanta. When the medical staff discovered his racial identity, they transferred him across the street to the ward designated for African American patients. It was too late for the doctors to save his life. White noted that neither his father nor his family "objected to the fact that his possession of a small amount of Negro blood caused him to be put in the 'Negro' ward"; however, he was critical of the fact that "that ward, being designated 'for Negroes,' was vastly inferior to the accommodations for whites."[51] Throughout his career, White rejected the premise of "separate but equal." He understood that his father's preventable death was part of a broader pattern. White compared his father's story to that of Juliette Derricotte—a Fisk University dean who, after being injured in a car accident in Georgia, was denied timely treatment at a local hospital and died on the way to a facility designated for Black patients. "Had she had immediate hospitalization," White noted, "she could have lived, the doctors agreed."[52]

On the night that his father died, White recounted how a screen was placed around his bed. While the voices of visitors from the Black community "filled the large, dingy room with sound," White was alarmed that suddenly there emerged a group of white singers who sang a "hymn and intoned whining prayers, smug in their sense of racial superiority." "I could not in that atmosphere," White recounted, "and in that moment as my father lay there dying stomach insincere and hypocritical talk of a heavenly father for all mankind by members of a race which denied even decent hospitalization to one I loved," and he asked them to leave the room, after which they insulted him.[53] The tragedy of White's father's death—and the jarring confrontation with ostensibly sympathetic mourning hymns delivered by prejudiced visitors—exposed the kinds of failures within the medical system, and the limits of white compassion, that White dedicated a portion of his career and his fiction writing to addressing.

White's commitment to Black success in the medical professions, the desegregation of medical care, and a sense of the social causes of ill-health emerged at the foreground of his 1924 novel *The Fire in the Flint*. In this novel, White both critiqued the medical system and expressed an alternative vision for empowering forms of professional medical care. *Fire in the Flint* initially sets up readers' expectations for a plot centered on upward mobility, respectability, and assimilation through medical-professional practice, only to subvert these assumptions by transforming into a sustained interrogation of racial injustice within the medical system. Although in the novel White initially is optimistic about African Americans' entrance into the medical professions, he ultimately offers a searingly pessimistic critique of the social conditions that compromise both professionalism and collective health. In other words, while the novel's beginning foregrounds the protagonist's pursuit of professional success, it ultimately privileges his larger role within the community and the impediments that he faces in this broader context. White noted in an essay that early twentieth-century African American novelists tended either to portray characters from the masses or to write "novels of ambition" featuring exceptional individuals. In the latter category, he observed, "some, if not all, of the principal Negro characters seek definitely to rise above their levels, fired by ambition common to all human nature."[54] *Fire in the Flint* is partially a novel of ambition, but it also functions as a fundamental critique of race relations by shifting its focus from individual career ambitions to an institutional critique of the medical system. In the novel, the physician protagonist, Ken, returns to the South, but at first decides to practice medicine rather than engage in more social and political efforts in an attempt to escape the "race problem" as it is defined in the novel. However, the inherently political nature of his practice makes it impossible for him to avoid it. The narrative unfolds as both a tragedy of thwarted professional ambition and a critique of the social forces jeopardizing Black health, as revealed through the minor characters Ken encounters and the patients he strives to heal.

Fire in the Flint opens with Ken's expectations for success in his medical practice. In his office, Ken "fingered with almost loving tenderness" his equipment and experienced an "inward contentment." [55] Yet his optimism about potential economic success is starkly juxtaposed with the pervasive sickness, suffering, and injury he expects to confront. White writes that Ken "hoped and expected" his clean white index cards would soon be "filled with the names of innumerable sick people he was treating." [56] Although such hopes make sense economically, they raise ethical and social questions. When Ken tells his brother, Bob, that he returned to the South to make more money,[57] he later adds, almost as an afterthought, that he also wanted to serve his community: "I can do more good here, both for myself and for the colored people." For Bob, however, Ken's narrow focus on economic gain reveals a disregard for urgent political issues, as exemplified when Bob remarks, "you don't go out of the house unless you are hurrying to give somebody a pill or a dose of medicine."[58] Bob sees professionalism as unnecessarily tempering efforts to directly combat racial injustice.

White contends, however, that the medical profession is not separable from questions of racism and resistance but is in fact fundamentally intertwined with them. Ken's love interest, Jane, tells him that if "one of your patients had a cancer, you wouldn't advise him to use Christian Science in treating it, would you? . . . No, you wouldn't! You'd operate! And that's just what the colored people and the white people of the South have got to do . . . If they don't, then this thing they call the race problem is going to grow so big it's going to consume the South and America."[59] By evoking an "operation" as remedying the "race problem" through the analogy of an illness with deadly, metastasizing effects, Jane articulates a vision of medical care that is inherently political. As opposed to associations with the alternative of Christian Science—a creed that eschews professional medical treatment—this figuration grounds racial protest in the power of scientific medicine.

At the same time, the association between the "race problem" and ill-health turns out to be more than metaphorical. Throughout the novel, White underscores that racial violence directly produces physical injury and illness. Although Ken's work initially inspires high hopes, his practice forces him to confront patients he cannot save. When Bud Ware, a Pullman porter, is shot and left with only a few hours to live, Ken administers an opiate to ease his suffering. As Bud dies, Ken feels himself slowly drawn into the "race problem."[60] When Nancy Ware, Bud's wife, is attacked by the KKK, and Ken tries to help her in his role as a physician, he becomes imbued with precisely the kind of "furious rage" against the perpetuators of this crime that, it should be noted, Bob had earlier suggested his professionalism would necessarily work to suppress.[61]

The commitment to medical care as a form of protest is met in the novel with additional challenges. In the early twentieth century, Black physicians were sometimes mistrusted by Black patients out of fear of professional incompetence. As William Edward Burghardt Du Bois observed, "at first it would seem natural for Negroes to patronize Negro merchants, lawyers, and physicians, from a sense of pride and as a protest against race feeling among whites. When, however, we come to think further, we can see many hindrances. If a child is sick, the father wants a good physician; he knows plenty of good white physicians; he knows nothing of the skill of the black doctor, for the black doctor has no opportunity to exercise his skill . . ." .[62] In *Fire in the Flint*, this kind of mistrust means that Ken does not receive the "flood of patients" he anticipated.[63] When Emma Bradley, a family friend, falls ill, she declares she does not want a Black physician to treat her. After the therapies of a white doctor, Bennet, prove ineffective, Ken is called upon—but, as in Chesnutt's *Marrow* with the initial resistance to William's care for Dodie—only when no other white physicians are available. White situates this scene within a wider historical context, noting that the community of "Central City had been impressed upon them by three hundred years of slavery and the so-called freedom after the Emancipation Proclamation that no Negro doctor, however talented, was quite as good as a white one."[64] In this way, White suggests that a deep-seated mistrust of medical authority is a result of a history of slavery rather than a deficiency in modern Black physicians' skills.

In addition, other obstacles to Ken's professional success arise in the scene of care for Emma. White suggests that the low proportion of African American physicians—a result of prejudiced forms of gatekeeping—can lead to unnecessary conflict among them. When Ken asks Dr. Williams for assistance with the operation on Emma, Ken realizes his dependency on Williams, because "no white doctor would assist a Negro surgeon."[65] But Williams, an established physician, objects with an air of affront—noting that he is "*the* coloured physician of Central City"—and resents being asked to assist a younger man.[66] White emphasizes the need for a humanitarian and civic duty in medicine that transcends competition for status. Yet such competition becomes inevitable in the face of professional exclusion that allows only token representation. However, while the doctors eventually agree to operate together, White shows how the relentless assault of white supremacism continues to threaten Black health. Although Williams eventually agrees to help and Emma's life is saved, the success of one operation remains a partial remedy. The scene concludes with a reminder that the prejudice nearly costing Emma her life will continue to degrade the quality of care many patients receive. When Ken attempts to confirm his diagnosis with Bennet, the latter responds with prejudiced medical theories.

As a result of this inequitable context, *Fire in the Flint*, like *Marrow*, concludes with a scene of cross-racial medical care that subverts melodramatic expectations. When one patient, Mary Ewing, falls ill, her father declares he would rather see her dead than have an African American doctor treat her. However, Mary's mother insists on treatment, and Ken reflects, "The color and race of the surgeon had been almost forgotten in the strange circumstances . . . Race prejudice is a funny thing! When it came to recognizing a Negro outside of menial service, there came the rub . . ." He adds, "in a matter of life and death like Ewing's case, they forgot prejudice."[67] White echoes Chesnutt's critique in *Marrow* and "The Ideal Nurse" that white Americans would consult Black physicians and trained nurses only when absolutely necessary, even as they regularly exploited forms of less professionalized labor. Ultimately, Ken's care for Mary is accepted solely because her condition is life-threatening. White forces readers to ask whether, in a segregated—and therefore inherently unequal—medical system, cross-racial care can truly ameliorate the "race problem" in the first place. There is even a suggestion that Ken contemplates substituting care for violence as a form of retribution. The interplay between care and violence in *Fire in the Flint* echoes Chesnutt's *Marrow*, where William at first considers withholding care from Dodie. Throughout the novel, Ken increasingly comes to ponder whether violence might be a viable response to racial injustice, and in the final scene, as Ken tends to Mary, this fighting spirit emerges prominently. Confronted with the possibility of retribution against "that race which had done irreparable, irremediable harm to him," Ken briefly entertains the notion, "Why not let her serve as a vicarious sacrifice for that race?"[68] Although White ultimately has Ken reject such a sacrifice, he still privileges a kind of combative posture insofar as he uses this scene, on the verge of tipping into violence, to unsettle liberal fantasies that individual acts of compassionate healing would serve as resolutions to entrenched injustices.

White's emphasis on this kind of "fighting spirit" is encapsulated in his description of Ken's smile in this scene. When he momentarily stops administering medication to Mary, her mother misinterprets his smile as one marking progress in saving her daughter's life, yet White reveals it to be a "hard smile," formed in the fleeting moment in which Ken fantasizes about letting his patient die.[69] Whereas the novel begins with Ken's "smile of satisfaction"[70] in his new office, reflecting happiness about his career, by the end of the novel, his hardened smile echoes the "fighting spirit" embodied by his brother Bob. In fact, in a parallel plot line, Bob commits suicide to escape a white mob who is attacking him, and Bob has on his face as he dies a "sardonic smile as though he laughed in death at cheating the howling pack of the satisfaction of killing him."[71] Ken's terse smile, like Bob's, is a direct response to white supremacist violence. Rather than expressing satisfaction in providing life-saving medical care, this smile is about the possibility of revenge.

Ultimately, Ken's care for Mary is accepted only because her case is life-threatening, yet his professional ethics and willingness to risk his own safety are violently repaid. Shortly after saving Mary, Ken is killed after being accused falsely of sexual violence. Although the life-threatening nature of his patient's condition challenges the logic of segregation temporarily, the care provided by Ken does not produce any meaningful social change, and professional medical skill is met with punishment rather than reciprocal compassion or understanding. Ken saves Mary's life, and White implicitly concedes that the "fighting spirit" encouraged by Bob must not be directed against an innocent, vulnerable patient. Yet, as with William's treatment of Dodie in *Marrow*, Ken's care for a white child does not establish a path toward better race relations either. In White's understanding, there could be no individual resolutions to social problems such as segregation and medical violence, and in fact acts of individual care unaccompanied by social change could detract attention away from issues that were national in scope.

This commitment to critique that White probed in *Fire in the Flint* animated his reform work. Because medicine is fundamentally about alleviating suffering, White recognized it could have served as a potent challenge to segregation and was disappointed in instances in which it did not. In an October 1936 letter written in his role as NAACP Secretary, White addressed a New York County Medical Society regarding an invitation from the Southern Medical Association that welcomed "white members in good standing of their state medical societies" to its annual meeting in Baltimore. White urged the New York County Medical School to discourage its members from attendance, writing, "We know you agree that if there is any one field of human endeavor in which race prejudice should be actively opposed, it should be in the great profession of healing the sick."[72]

White resisted the notion of "separate but equal" in medicine throughout his career. In a 1947 article in the *New York Herald Tribune*, he praised Dr. W. Montague Cobb's "Medical Care and the Plight of the Negro," published in *Crisis*, which addressed the professional barriers faced by many Black physicians. White noted that barred from both public and private hospitals, they were unable to treat their patients. Compounding the effects of this discrimination, African Americans were routinely accused of having inherently higher morbidity and mortality rates, as a result of perceived biological factors. White argued that earlier studies of African American health were predicated on the assumption of "separate but equal" facilities, and he admired Cobb for challenging that notion. Desegregation, White contended, had to be complete, and individual interracial hospitals were insufficient to remedy national racial inequities. Thinking alongside Cobb's argument, he maintained that "so-called 'interracial'" hospitals in cities like New York, Cleveland, and Chicago—often built with the support of philanthropic investments—were typically established in lower-quality facilities with obsolete infrastructures and fewer resources. In his view, these institutions fostered a false sense of progress among white Americans while in fact further perpetuating segregation. Instead of such a scenario, White advocated for "the integration of all doctors, specialists, and nurses irrespective of race, creed, color, or national origin in hospital systems generally."[73]

Later, White opposed a bill to create a Black veterans' hospital at Booker T. Washington's birthplace in Virginia—a proposal sponsored by the government. In 1948, White participated in a committee meeting convened by Senator Wayne Morse on this issue.[74] One proponent read aloud a letter from Booker T. Washington's daughter, Portia Washington Pittman, who argued that the hospital would serve as an "inspiration" to Black veterans.[75] The vice president of the Booker T. Washington Birthplace Memorial added that, since most Black veterans lived in segregated regions with limited access to medical care, the hospital would help remedy that problem. White countered this point by reminding the subcommittee that "separate but equal" was a legal fiction and that a segregated hospital would "give federal sanction to the furtherance of substandard medical treatment for Negro veterans and would place the stamp of Federal approval on segregation."[76] Although supporters invoked Booker T. Washington's legacy, White argued that Washington himself would have opposed the hospital, viewing it as a result of segregation. White further maintained that even white liberal opinion was turning against segregation, and that creating such a hospital would represent a major regression. In 1951, White's position prevailed when the legislative proposal was rejected by the House of Representatives.[77]

White argued that equality was impossible when a white-dominated medical profession largely barred Black doctors from working in many hospitals, including Harlem Hospital even though, as White noted in his memoir *A Man Called White* (1948), many of them had trained in "top-flight medical schools." As White suggested, this was evidence that the "poison of race prejudice, and even more, of ignorance about the Negro's potentialities, had penetrated the North."[78] Furthermore, drawing on his personal experience and reform work, White observed that patients "were treated with such scant efficiency at Harlem Hospital that the situation had produced a folk saying: 'When any member of your family goes to Harlem Hospital, telephone the undertaker.'"[79] White had worked with surgeon Louis Wright to present research into the subpar conditions at Harlem Hospital to Mayor John F. Hylan, which led to calls for investigations of the complaints and public hearings. The only resolution, they noted, was for New York City to "abandon its unwritten law" against the admission of qualified Black "doctors, specialists, and nurses to New York City hospitals." As White would insist upon throughout his career, desegregation had to occur immediately rather than gradually. After Wright, in collaboration with White, the North

Harlem Medical Association and the NAACP, exposed racial discrimination at Harlem Hospital, a compromise was offered to establish a hospital to be staffed entirely by African American physicians. But Wright questioned whether accepting a Jim Crow institution—no matter how well-equipped— was preferable to complete integration. White paraphrased Wright, noting "the chief advantage to Negro doctors of opportunity to serve in hospitals was that of learning and competing with the best men in the field, and that acceptance of segregated training would fix forever upon the Negro a differential of training and experience. This, in turn, would do harm to the Negro doctors' patients and perpetuate a higher morbidity and mortality rate among Negroes." He concluded: "Second-class status must never be accepted, however long and difficult the attainment of first-class opportunity might be."[80] For White, such a hospital would not resolve the challenges physicians faced in acquiring expertise and would in fact further entrench segregation.

In a 1952 article in *The Chicago Defender*, White recounted an event at New York's Statler Hotel where leaders in education, civil rights, public affairs, and medicine celebrated the achievements of Wright, including his contributions to health reform. Among the honorees were Eleanor Roosevelt and the "Kentucky-born president of the American College of Surgeons, Dr. Henry W. Cave, who fought and smashed the color bar in the most eminent and professional societies . . ." White noted that Wright, as chief of surgery at New York's interracial Harlem Hospital, had made significant contributions to scientific research; yet, White remarked, "even were I informed enough to write about science, I would prefer writing about the man himself." Although Wright could have charged high fees for his services, he chose instead to make personal sacrifices for science. White celebrated Wright for opposing the exclusion of African Americans from the medical profession, admiring his assertion that "segregation in itself is and always would be inequality." Changes to the profession would have to be sweeping and immediate rather than gradual and incremental. In *Fire in the Flint*, White had implicitly argued for the importance of Black representation within the profession, but this had been part of the task of contributing to the broader aims of desegregation and combatting prejudice within medicine. Though many physicians saw Wright's rejection of any measures possible to increase professional representation as unrealistic, Wright insisted on total equality within and beyond the medical professions rather than increased representation alone, and White affirmed this strategy.[81]

Demanding sweeping social transformation and pursuing complete equality would necessitate a shift away from reductive melodramas of compassionate care. White had begun to express as much in his account of the hypocritical hymn singing by white visitors at the hospital where his father died, and in the *Fire in the Flint* with the failures of white compassion and the privileging of a "fighting spirit" in response. In fact, throughout his career he would remain attuned to cultural representations of medicine that challenged reductive melodramas of care. This becomes evident in his *Chicago Defender* review of a film released years after the publication of *The Fire in the Flint*, the medical drama *No Way Out* (1950),[82] which like *Fire in the Flint* refused to appeal reductively to cross-racial harmony. *No Way Out's* dramatic tension centers on physician Dr. Luther Brooks, played by Sidney Poitier in his debut, who provides care for an injured, white supremacist prisoner Ray and his brother, Johnny at a city hospital. After Johnny dies of medical complications, Ray attempts to frame Luther for his death. In the film's climax, Ray shoots Luther, wounding him severely, while Ray's own already-injured leg is further torn, causing him excruciating pain. In his agony, Ray exclaims, "Who cares? Who cares about me? Does anybody care about me . . . if I'm bleeding . . . burning . . . Nobody cares about Ray Biddle." Although this reference to care is not explicitly about medicine, it resonates with the film's overall emphasis on medical themes and specifically the way Ray sees Luther as a threat rather than a respected professional. Defying Ray's expectations, Luther saves Ray's life by using Ray's gun to tie off a bandage on his leg, thereby stopping the bleeding. In so doing he turns an instrument of violence into a mechanism of healing. Yet what is crucial is this act of healing is not portrayed as purely compassionate, or at least not in any overly rosy sense. As Luther consigns Ray to a future of suffering and guilt while assuring him of survival, his tone is menacing and his facial expression enraged, as the film subverts any audience expectations for complete empathy or closure in the face of ongoing, injurious injustices.

Recognizing the critical commentary on conventional racial melodrama made in the film, White praised *No Way Out's* "courage and clarity of vision" in confronting "racial bigots," noting that although some might claim the story is overdrawn in certain episodes, such criticism was unfounded. For White, the film was melodramatic, to be sure, but in fact the melodrama was so potent that "the spectator can hardly breathe because of excitement," as White alluded specifically to the film's ending.[83] The melodrama, in White's view, was meant to unsettle viewers and make them uncomfortable, much like the effect of Ken's ambiguous smile over his patient Mary's body in *Fire in the Flint*. According to White, privileging individual, melodramatic scenes of compassionate care, much like the support of only individual Black or interracial medical institutions, threatened to detract attention from the need for a fundamental overhaul of the very foundations of segregation and entrenched forms of medical racism in American society.

Rewriting Psychiatry

Throughout the early twentieth century, persistent challenges to the "separate but equal" doctrine affecting medical care would be met with white supremacist resistance. Writing at a key moment of national efforts toward desegregation in the mid-twentieth century, novelist and literary critic Ralph Ellison, then living in New York City, confronted a segregated and violent medical system and proposed professional medical alternatives. Like Chesnutt and White, Ellison portrayed scenes of cross-racial care that were riddled by tension and violence, while emphasizing the need for critiquing medical injustices. Like Chesnutt and White, too, Ellison positioned Black representation within the medical profession as one component of combatting these injustices but also insisted that representation needed to be paired with alternative kinds of medical institutions, policies, and practices. Ellison was particularly interested in psychiatry, which raised a host of questions about both the institutional shape of medical care and the nexus of psychological and racial forces affecting patients. Questions of psychiatry and race profoundly influenced his life, reform work, and fictional output, and these concerns reached their most extensive articulation in *Invisible Man* (1952).

Ellison observed that patients experiencing psychological distress could be oppressed both by the stigma of mental illness and by racism. In his era, psychiatry was minimally regulated. Widespread fear of those suffering from mental illness led to its criminalization. This was an age of frequent lobotomies, electroconvulsive therapy, involuntary admissions, and vague diagnostic classifications.[84] But psychiatric violence was particularly acute when it intersected with racial prejudice. Since the nineteenth century, a white-dominated medical profession had grossly mischaracterized African Americans' psychological suffering, ignoring the harmful impacts of racial oppression on mental health while labeling resistance to it as pathological. Mississippi physician Samuel Cartwright, cloaking racial ideologies in scientific language, coined the diagnosis "drapetomania" to describe what he claimed was a condition that caused enslaved African Americans to flee captivity.[85] These kinds of theories did not end with emancipation but continued into the twentieth century. In 1913, for instance, psychiatrist Arrah B. Evarts, writing in *The Psychoanalytical Review*, discussed "dementia precox" in language that echoed Cartwright's assertions: Evarts claimed that "bondage in reality was a wonderful aid" and that freedom, conversely, led to mental decline.[86] Meanwhile, as psychiatrist Frederic Wertham observed, African American populations were often "not allowed the luxury of neurosis . . . The official view is that they are just unhappy, or they need housing, or they feel downtrodden."[87] While frequently classified as suffering mental illnesses based on egregious biological myths, genuine forms of psychological suffering simultaneously went under-diagnosed and untreated.

For Ellison, the Lafargue Mental Hygienic Clinic promised to address these injustices. Named for the French Marxist doctor and social reformer Paul Lafargue, the interracial clinic provided low-cost psychiatric care to Harlem patients from 1946 to 1958. Its founder, Wertham, employed a form of social psychiatry that prioritized understanding how racial prejudice—compounded by economic exploitation—affected mental health,[88] and Ellison worked closely with Wertham to promote the clinic. Their collaboration began during World War II, when Ellison, having resisted the draft under Jim Crow conditions, encountered Wertham through a meeting organized by novelist Richard Wright. A letter from Wertham, which justified Ellison's draft exemption on psychiatric grounds, laid the foundation for Ellison's enduring professional alliance with Wertham, and his efforts to raise awareness about the Lafargue Clinic.[89]

Critics have noted Ellison's critique of psychiatric violence and exploitation, but, as his work with the Lafargue Clinic points toward, he also grappled with specific ways it could be reformed. Shelly Eversley, in discussing forms of psychiatric harm in Ellison's work, argues that in *Invisible Man*, Ellison "imagines madness as a radical break from an incarcerating power," as the narrator "finds himself in a psychiatric hospital because he defies authority and by the end of the novel he comes to believe his freedom and his humanity depends on that defiance."[90] The notion that Ellison offers a rejection of psychiatric labels and disciplinary structures has often been predicated on a sense that he understands psychiatric classifications of psychological conditions to be unfounded. J. Bradford Campbell suggests that Ellison treats the diagnosis of mental illness as arbitrary, arguing that instead of accepting mental illness as a fixed reality, Ellison depicts neurosis as very ambiguous, complicating the traditional "divide between sanity and insanity itself."[91] As Cera Smith has demonstrated, Ellison explores both the psychological and physiological violence inflicted on patients by medical authorities, noting that *Invisible Man* portrays "social invisibility, not as a metaphor but as an embodied, somatic state through racializing violence" and argues that "racist doctors injure the protagonist's brain through electro-shock torture, disrupting his cognition and sympathetic nervous system."[92] In *Invisible Man* Ellison exposes the subjective nature of psychiatric classifications and critiques medical violence. But, at the same time, Ellison was drawn to the kinds of psychiatric insights offered by the Lafargue Clinic, viewing them as potentially productive, and throughout his writing, Ellison reoriented readers to the possibilities of psychiatry, when wielded through a radically reimagined understanding. La Marr Jurelle Bruce's argument for a "critical ambivalence" toward psychiatry is instructive here: while he suggests it is essential to draw on "antipsychiatry's attention to racism ... and other pernicious ideologies that have effected and affected mainstream psychiatry," he suggests, it is also true that "many psychiatric clients and consumers find healing and even empowerment through clinical intervention."[93] Informed by this kind of ambivalence, Ellison engaged with psychiatric authority in ways that unsettled its harmful manifestations while also privileging the liberatory possibilities that it could unlock.

Throughout his writing, Ellison elaborated on the connections between psychology and the effects of white hatred within the social order. In his essay "Beating that Boy" (1945), he suggested the United States was a nation of "ethical schizophrenics" and that white Americans' "unwillingness to resolve the conflict in keeping with his democratic ideals has compelled the white American, figuratively, to force the Negro down into the deeper level of his consciousness ... down into the province of the psychiatrist and the artist, from whence spring the lunatic's fancy and the work of art."[94] Here, Ellison suggested that white hate is predicated on a dangerous kind of madness that surpasses the recognition of hard truths about race relations. In addition, in "Richard Wright's Blues" (1945), Ellison argued that families must "adjust the child to the Southern milieu," a process that can develop into a "defence mechanism" to prevent the child "from whirling away from the undifferentiated mass of his people into the unknown, symbolized in its most abstract form by insanity, and most concretely by lynching."[95] Through this parallel construction, Ellison contended that both violence and mental illness are responses to the unknown, shaped by a landscape of haunting uncertainty produced by white supremacist hatred. In fact, this hatred was so pervasive that it was often necessary, in Ellison's psychoanalytical understanding, to "flee hysterically into the sleep of violence or the coma of apathy..."[96]

This state resonates with the kind of psychological state Ellison described elsewhere as "nowhere," a mood marked by haunting uncertainty. In his essay "Harlem is Nowhere" (1948), Ellison inquired of the typical Lafargue Clinic patient, "what is the psychological character of the scene in which he dwells; how describe the past which he drags to this scene, and what is the future toward which he stumbles and becomes confused?" For Ellison, Harlem—with its crime and crumbling infrastructures—was a nightmare "indistinguishable from the distorted images that can appear in dreams." Yet he noted, this "was no dream" but a "reality." Harlem's very environment, he argued, seemed to symbolically possess a distinct psychological character, and in fact, this environment directly led to psychological suffering in its inhabitants. Consistent with the Lafargue Clinic's mission, Ellison called for the treatment of psychological distress—particularly the kind that had come to be medically recognized—in ways that attended to these environmental conditions.[97]

Access to quality psychiatric care was crucial. In "Harlem is Nowhere," Ellison contended that the Lafargue Clinic was "perhaps the most successful attempt in the nation to provide psychotherapy to the underprivileged" and one of the few institutions offering effective psychiatric care to African American patients. He regarded the clinic's work as indispensable at a time when therapeutic options were severely limited. Ellison argued that the response to discrimination in Harlem could devolve into "hysterical forms of religion" and addiction as African Americans remained unable to "participate fully in the therapy which the white American achieves through patriotic ceremonies and by identifying himself with American wealth and power." By filling the void created by insufficient mental health resources and a distorted, racialized therapeutic culture, the Lafargue Clinic provided a necessary counterbalance. Ellison maintained that whereas white Americans could find psychological relief in national symbols and patriotic celebrations, African Americans—aware of the false promises of American democracy—were instead unsettled by the hypocrisy underlying these practices.

For Ellison, addressing psychological suffering required transforming formal, institutional psychiatry. In his unpublished notes for "Harlem is Nowhere," Ellison insisted on the importance of enabling African Americans to participate more fully "in the institutional life of the U.S.," explaining that "one of the major psychological functions of a social institution is that of protecting the citizen against the irrational forces of the world. The right to participate brings more with it than the badge of belonging; it is also an armor against anxiety."[98] This principle applied specifically to the psychiatric establishment, which, Ellison argued, needed to protect African American mental health through institutional channels. Ellison described the Lafargue Clinic as providing an essential resource within an otherwise compromised medical system: before it was established, he noted, African Americans "who required treatment had nowhere to turn." Although the title of his essay "Harlem is Nowhere" employs "nowhere" as a metaphysical descriptor of a state of despair, in Ellison's notes for the essay the term specifically denotes the absence of viable mental health services available to Harlem patients. In these notes, Ellison further observed that "New York's mental institutions do not accept" Black patients "unless they have reached a point where they require confinement." And very often," he continued, "when Negroes seek the help of private psychiatrists, they find the psychiatrist cannot help them because the psychiatrist is afflicted by the same conditions that attack the patient. As for Negro psychiatrists, as the result of economic and social discrimination, there are about eight in the country. Even when he sought scientific help, the Negro found himself in a maze."[99] Ellison argued that racial prejudice had distorted a predominantly white profession into a state of near madness, leaving many patients with confusion rather than effective care.

More broadly, Ellison suggested that race relations in the US had obscured and distorted a sense of the nature of the realities of psychological suffering, and that in reckoning with these realities, one could better protect one's own well-being. He noted that Harlem patients were "not unaware that the conditions of their lives demanded new definitions of terms like . . . sanity and insanity" and he sought to dispel the myth that African Americans were inherently prone to mental illness. He recognized that the need for the Lafargue Clinic was "chronic" not because the mental troubles of its patients were unique, but because harsh living conditions amplified any state of "psychological dispossession" to an extreme degree.[100] In emphasizing these concrete, material realities, Ellison grounded his discussion of mental health in the environment. In addition, Ellison took an introspective turn by suggesting that in redefining sanity and insanity in ways that attended to racial oppression, he could shield himself from trauma. In the wake of ongoing racism in the United States, Ellison observed that one might feel compelled to acknowledge the reality of "white oppression." As he put it, "So, like you, I actually live in a state that is neither sane nor insane, neither in the South nor in the North; neither in the US in which other Americans live, nor out of it; it is a state in which two times two never quite equals four, and in which citizenship has never meant equality. And, like you, in order not to clutter my life by constantly contemplating the painful, I have concluded that we live in a state of Nowhere."[101] Recognizing that one lives in a "state of Nowhere" served as a survival strategy, becoming a means to escape the irrationality of racial prejudice and its painful effects. Although Ellison noted that "Nowhere" was neither "sane" nor "insane," he maintained that coming to understand himself as being "nowhere"—a realization spurred by his appreciation for the mission integral to the Lafargue Clinic's underground psychiatry—was an attempt to protect his own sanity.[102]

Ellison recognized that while "insanity" was a medical reality, it had to be re-conceptualized in ways that did not reinforce racial prejudice but instead actively subverted it. Ellison was critical of how a mainstream, white-dominated psychiatric profession offered supposedly expert resolutions to psychological traumas without accounting for the effects of racism. In his essay "The Shadow and the Act" (1948), Ellison discussed the film *Home of the Brave*, in which a psychiatrist tells a soldier that his "hysterical paralysis is like that of any other soldier who has lived when his friends have died;" the soldier is declared cured and seen walking away, prepared to open a bar and restaurant with a white veteran.[103] However, Ellison stressed that this scene evaded the "racial element in the motivation of his guilt." The soldier had wished his friend dead after being called a racial slur, and soon after, his friend was killed by a sniper's bullet. "What happens," Ellison asked, "to the racial element in the motivation of his guilt?" The psychiatrist's dismissal—noting that the soldier is "like everyone else"—exemplifies a seemingly neutral and universalizing but in fact deeply prejudiced approach to medical care. Because of this kind of thinking, Ellison argued that traumas produced by racist aggression exceeded the explanatory power of white-dominated psychiatric expertise. Under Jim Crow, Ellison noted, "psychiatry is not, I'm afraid, the answer. The soldier suffers from concrete acts, not hallucinations."[104] As Badia Sahar Ahad has shown, Ellison rejected conventional psychoanalysis's focus on individual dynamics, instead positing that mental illness originates in the "social order."[105] Ellison's commentary in "The Shadow and the Act" correspondingly places questions of racial justice at the center of a consideration of psychology.

While in "The Shadow and the Act," Ellison was driven to reject psychiatric explanations for certain kinds of suffering altogether, Ellison's commitment to reforming psychiatry is extensively elaborated upon in *Invisible Man*. Early in the novel, the narrator asks, "But what did *I* do to be so blue?"[106] and Ellison addresses this question through a perspective informed by progressive psychiatry. The kind of melancholy experienced by the narrator has been taken up in psychoanalytical criticism. For instance, Anne Anlin Cheng has turned to *Invisible Man* to ask, "Can there be a progressive politics that recognizes, rather than denies, the raced subject's melancholic desires?" She argues that such a politics would require "neither dismissing nor sentimentalizing minority desires," but rather understanding the "political potentials of melancholic subjectivity."[107] Psychoanalytical interpretations of fiction risk stigmatizing the populations characters represent, but when psychology is understood as being shaped by racism and resistance, representations of psychological pain, even the kinds understood formally in psychiatric terms, become recognizable as responses to socially inflicted injustices.

Ellison's strategy of reworking psychiatric insights in ways that account for social conditions becomes evident in the scene of the Golden Day pub, where "shell-shocked" veterans from a nearby asylum gather, and where their madness is depicted as revelatory, in contrast to Norton, a college trustee who assumes the role of the benevolent white protector but is portrayed as helplessly deluded. As a doctor committed to psychological understanding and neurology, the character of the physician-veteran exemplifies how Ellison reclaims professional medical perspectives to address the traumas inflicted by racial violence. When Norton faints, the physician-veteran speaks "very professionally," as Ellison asserts the veteran character's medical authority even as he has been forced to assume the position of a patient.

He feels Norton's pulse, and advises, "Rest, rest . . . The clocks are all set back and the forces of destruction are rampant down below . . ." Although the injunction to "rest" sounds therapeutic, it is a medical prescription tinged with an ominous prophecy. The atmosphere has a clarifying effect on the perception of race relations, as when Norton collapses, he appears as a "formless white death . . . a death which had been there all the time and which had now revealed itself in the madness of the Golden Day."[108] At the Golden Day pub, rather than administering violent electric shocks, the veterans articulate revelations about race relations in the United States that have the potential to shock their listeners. The asylum patients' madness emerges from suffering, and comes to proliferate profound insights, as they realize it is white hate where irrationality truly resides. The vet-physician tells Norton, "To some, you are the great white father, to others the lyncher of souls, but for all, you are confusion come even into the Golden Day.[109]" When Norton experiences a "mild shock," one patron remarks, "this here Golden Day is enough to shock anybody."[110] Meanwhile, the Golden Day crowd engages in a collective mode of therapy based on catharsis, joy, conversation, and the "healing touch" of Hester—a bartender described as both a "therapist" and a "humanitarian."[111] The "confusion" of the Golden Day crowd, unlike that of Norton, is predicated on sharp insights into the psychological effects of racial oppression.

Ellison devoted particular attention to challenging the myths bolstered by a white-dominated psychiatric establishment in critiquing conventional understandings of anger. In this sense, *Invisible Man* resonates with forms of progressive psychiatric thought from the mid-twentieth century that revised entrenched racist discourses about anger. As Jonathan Metzl notes,[112] in 1968 psychiatrists Walter Bromberg and Franck Simon published "The 'Protest' Psychosis" in the *Archives of General Psychiatry*, arguing that the "stress" of advocating for civil rights and the "nationalist fervor of Africo-Asian nations . . . [had] stimulated specific reactive psychoses in American Negroes."[113] They maintained that this "protest psychosis" became visible when individuals were convicted of crimes—and that it originally emerged from civil rights protesters' denial of the "values" of white people. This theory represented a particularly egregious instantiation of an ideology pervasive in US culture and medicine. But it has been persistently challenged. In the 1940s, for instance, psychiatrist Benjamin Karpman encouraged his Howard University medical students to consider how racism could produce psychic distress by analyzing Richard Wright's *Native Son* (1940) and speculating about the "social and economic factors" underlying Bigger Thomas's mental anguish. One student, for instance, suggested that Bigger might have killed Mary, a wealthy white woman, because of "ignorance, family influences, gangs, poor environmental conditions" and " a society that is warped with discrimination and prejudice..."[114] Later in the twentieth century, in *Black Rage* (1968), psychiatrists William H. Grier and Price M. Cobbs argued that what they called "black rage" was not confined to a "few 'extremists,'" but was a widespread condition engendered by prejudice.[115] Although they entertained Freudian speculations involving "castration anxiety" and "counterphobic functioning," they insisted for instance that the anger of a patient was most "encompassed within a larger social dynamic which was set in motion before his birth,"[116] an insight that echoed throughout their work as a whole.

Ellison participated in a similar tradition of thought, resonating with Karpman as well as with Grier and Cobbs by arguing that anger, even the kind that can be understood in psychiatric terms, is often a response to racial prejudice. This revised medical understanding of anger is first expressed in *Invisible Man*'s preface, where the narrator recounts accidentally being bumped into by a man on the street. This man insulted him—and the narrator demands that he apologize. When he does not do so, the narrator attacks him and takes out a knife, preparing to slit the man's throat. Ellison suggests that the narrator's violent thoughts are spurred by hysteria: "Shouldn't he, for his own personal safety, have recognized my hysteria, my 'danger potential'?" In light of a deranged landscape of race relations produced by white hate, hysteria becomes a wholly fitting response. Diagnosing himself, the narrator describes his hysteria as real; it is "danger" that is put in quotation marks, and in fact Ellison refers to only the *potential* for danger. The narrator is justifiably angry, but he is not truly dangerous. He carefully controls his rage. Alternatively, the narrator suggests that the man who bumps into him has lost control of his mind, as he is "lost in a dream world," and yet, he asks, "didn't he control that dream world—which, alas, is only too real!" Here, Ellison echoed "Harlem is Nowhere," in which he noted Harlem seemed full of "distorted images" appearing in dreams but that what appeared to be dreams were in fact realities that led to outbursts of anger. The man who has bumped into him is complicit in producing a violent kind of nightmare. The man is oblivious, but willfully so, and this willful oblivion causes others to suffer. When the narrator admits he was the "irresponsible one," it is not because he should have left the man alone, but rather he claims, "I should have used my knife to protect the higher interests of society," channeling his anger into self-defense.[117] The narrator both controls his rage and regrets not acting on it as a response to a form of racial prejudice that is itself dangerous.

Later, in the Golden Day scene, the relationship between anger, mental illness, and racial prejudice is further elaborated upon. One character in the crowd exhibits a "glassy-eyed fury," illustrating how a particularly enlightened form of anger can sharpen perception. The physician-veteran explains that after being shunned by the army—despite his devoted care for wounded soldiers—his "hands so lovingly trained to master a scalpel yearn to caress a trigger."[118] The observation also resonates with Ellison's own defiant refusal to serve in a Jim Crow military under the auspices of Wertham's psychiatric authority. Here, however, a commitment to care has given way to violence. Norton explicitly dismisses the veteran's anger as insanity—declaring that "the man is as insane as the rest"[119] but alternatively, the narrator, tempted to label and dismiss the man as "crazy," instead experiences a "fearful satisfaction from hearing him talk as he had to a white man."[120] The narrator's point here is not to reject the presence of mental illness, but to gesture toward the need to understand that this psychological suffering is a response to injustice.

Ellison's depiction of anger is aligned specifically with the psychiatric concept of "free-floating hostility" that was theorized by Wertham at the Lafargue Clinic. Journalist Robert Bendiner observed that among Wertham's patients at Lafargue, "mental difficulties" were thought to arise from the "free-floating hostility" generated by severe social pressures—poverty, overcrowded living conditions, and persistent discrimination. Bendiner pondered, "What constitutes a constructive channel for such hostility, and isn't this approach likely to lead the clinic down political byways?"[121] Yet, in understanding that rage could be a response to racial violence, for Ellison, as for Wertham, it was precisely these "political byways" that would be critical to transforming professional psychiatry. In "Harlem is Nowhere," Ellison remarked that for Wertham, African Americans' "free-floating hostility" emerged from violence that produced a diffuse anger not targeted at any singular object. Ellison extended this idea in a version of "Harlem is Nowhere," initially intended to be published in *Magazine of the Year* when he suggested that such anger "with the world" sometimes "provokes mass responses, and the results are the spontaneous outbreaks called the Harlem riots of 1935 and 1943."[122] Rather than resisting the medicalization of anger, Ellison reformulated anger to account for its underlying social causes. In the Golden Day scene, this idea becomes aligned with the veterans' stance as they deliver "hostile speeches . . . at the top of their voices against the hospital," while also expressing a more general anger directed toward "the state" and even "the universe."[123] Akin to "free-floating hostility," the anger voiced by the patients at the Golden Day is targeted at the entire social fabric, of which the hospital is one part.

Ellison specifically elucidates the connections between racism and madness by situating individual psychological experiences within collective US histories. Some key strands of mid-twentieth-century psychiatry increasingly emphasized how large historical forces shape individual minds. For example, William H. Grier and Price M. Cobbs, who theorized about "black rage," recommended a therapeutic approach that included educating patients about the "racist history of the United States," thereby helping them understand that trauma often arises from historical forces beyond their control.[124] The effects of historical forces on individual minds would also be articulated by sociologist Calvin Hernton in his discussion of his 1974 novel *Scarecrow*. *Scarecrow* follows an emotionally disturbed protagonist who strangles his ex-wife, stores her body in a trunk, sets sail for England, and encounters a psychiatrist whose socially informed approach to mental illness centers critiques of racial prejudice.[125] While Hernton readily acknowledged the existence of illnesses such as schizophrenia, he was troubled by the dominance of Freudian explanations for them, which privileged individual and familial influences above sociopolitical and historical forces. He argued that, although psychoanalysis traditionally plumbed the depths of personal histories, effective therapy requires an understanding of a broader historical context. Hernton insisted that mental health discussions must incorporate a "historical and a sociological dimension" to "demystify the purely psychiatric or Freudian interpretation." As Hernton explained in his discussion of the genesis of *Scarecrow*, "I wanted to socially and historically locate what we refer to as schizophrenia . . . In treating the contemporary scene, all one is treating are symptoms. That treatment has to be informed with the weight of history."[126] In a way that anticipates these later explanations of the relationship between psychology and history, in *Invisible Man*, asylum patients offer incisive critiques of histories of race relations in the US to explain psychological phenomena. One individual asserts of Norton, "I should know my own grandfather! He's Thomas Jefferson and I'm his grandson." Early American history, in this context, is felt in deeply personal ways by the Golden Day characters and articulated as a foundation for critiques of the contemporary moment. This historical awareness is matched by sweeping, optimistic prophecies of change in the future. One Golden Day patient—a "student of history"—envisions historical progress through a visionary account: "the world moves in a circle like a roulette wheel. In the beginning, black is on top, in the middle epochs, white holds the odds, but soon Ethiopia shall stretch forth her noble wings!" Although this prophecy foretells a future in which "black" will be dominant, the speaker also anticipates a smaller, more immediate change: in "two years from now" he expects to care for his mother. By interweaving historical and individual time, his prophecy interweaves a long American history of racial violence and resistance with an account of personally, intimately felt experiences. Psychological trauma is passed down across generations. For Ellison, psychological suffering is positioned as a symptom of a violent, racist history, making it imperative to investigate and critically address that history as part of efforts to transform psychiatry and individuals' psychological lives.

In the Golden Day scene, Ellison envisions the potential of this subversive form of psychiatric wisdom—but that potential is foreclosed in the later factory hospital scene, where the narrator endures dehumanizing electroshock treatments after being injured at a paint factory, as Ellison suggests how a prejudiced profession fails to grasp the nature of psychological suffering. Ellison contrasts the narrator's complex, multifaceted psychological reality with the reductive simplifications imposed by the medical staff, who misunderstand his suffering, stigmatize his pain, and dehumanize him. The narrator observes, "I was sitting in a cold, white rigid chair and a man was looking at me out of a bright third eye that glowed from the center of his forehead."[127] Within this disciplinary, regimented, and "white" space, his initial belief—that he was in a hospital where care would ease his pain—proves tragically mistaken.[128] Instead, care is supplanted by violence when he overhears a discussion about a machine that "will produce the results of a prefrontal lobotomy without the negative effects of the knife."[129] This moment recalls the prologue in which a knife was invoked as the protagonist's potential means of protecting society from racial violence, though he ultimately resists using it; here, conversely, though no knife is used, violent shock treatments still serve to uphold a hierarchical racial order under the guise of care. In this context, the medical staff reduce the narrator to a threat. When a medical staff member inquires, "But what of his psychology?" another responds, "Absolutely of no importance! . . . The patient will live as he has to live, and with absolute integrity. Who could ask more? He'll experience no major conflict of motives, and what is even better, society will suffer no traumata on his account."[130] In this exchange, the medical staff perceives the narrator not as a suffering patient whose illness is a result of racial prejudice, but rather as a threat to a kind of "society" that they implicitly understand to be white. Readers, however, are privy to the narrator's insights. The narrator describes the relentless persistence of racial conflict, noting that "there was no avoiding the shock and I rolled with the agitated tide, out into the blackness," and he asks, "Where did my body end and the crystal and white world begin?"[131] He continues, "Thoughts evaded me, hiding in the vast stretch of clinical whiteness to which I seemed connected only by a scale of receding grays."[132] This psychological state, reminiscent of the "nowhere" Ellison described in "Harlem is Nowhere," reflects the confusion engendered by psychiatric racism, as the phrase "clinical whiteness" implicitly points to this white-dominated medical space from which he feels separated, while the reference to "receding grays" encapsulates the ambiguity and unsettling uncertainty of his experience as a patient. Later, he begins to wonder whether he was "just this blackness and bewilderment and pain" but then quickly distances himself from this understanding, refusing to internalize trauma entirely.[133] Through such sensory and subjective rhetoric, Ellison conveys how the medical team assaults not only the narrator's body via physical confinement but also his very sense of self, which he persistently resists through his very analysis of his treatment.

Extending the insights from the Golden Day scene regarding anger as a justified response to racial discrimination and violence, in the factory hospital scene Ellison presents a critically informed acceptance of anger as both a reasonable and necessary emotion. As the doctors administer electric shocks to him, the narrator describes his anger in self-reflective terms: "suddenly . . . I wanted to be angry, murderously angry. But somehow the pulse of current smashing through my body prevented me. Something had been disconnected. For though I had seldom used my capacities for anger and indignation, I had no doubt that I possessed them; and, like a man who knows that he must fight, whether angry or not, when called a son of a bitch, I tried to *imagine* myself angry—only to discover a deeper sense of remoteness. I was beyond anger."[134] Although potentially dangerous rage is understood as justified here, it remains frustratingly out of reach.

While the psychiatric profession could attempt to guard against patients' outbursts of anger, the narrator suggests, in a measured tone, that his anger is not only reasonable but desirable. This anger is deliberately suppressed by the doctors because they treat it as an individual pathology rather than a result of socially produced suffering. For the narrator, anger is a form of protest that is tragically being silenced.

Ellison's rendering of this moment of repressed resistance is part of his larger critique of conventional mental illness treatments. Recognizing the connection points between psychiatric authority and criminalization at an early moment, Ellison portrays psychiatric confinement in this scene as akin to imprisonment. The narrator, noting his head is surrounded by a piece of metal, likens his condition to that of a victim of an "electric chair"[135]: the doctors claim that their procedures effect personality changes reminiscent of "famous fairy-tale cases of criminals transformed into amiable fellows . . ." Yet the narrator remains confounded by this carceral logic being applied to his suffering: "Who am I? It was no good. I felt like a clown. Nor was I up to being both criminal and detective—though why criminal I didn't know."[136] The narrator refuses to answer the existential, deeply psychological question, *Who am I?* with any punishingly reductive answer.

Instead, readers are prodded to view the kind of psychiatric violence depicted in this scene, reaching its most absurd manifestation in the notion that the injured patient is a criminal, as foreclosing the earlier possibilities for psychiatric thought articulated within the Golden Day. By including these contrasting scenes that each implicate medical attitudes toward psychology, Ellison compels readers to consider how psychological distress is socially produced through racial injustice and how that dynamic can be either subverted or reinforced by medical authority.

Authors such as Chesnutt, White, and Ellison addressed racial injustices within modern medicine, as they envisioned revised forms of medical professionalism and knowledge capable of ameliorating them. Drawing on reform-minded medical knowledge, their work distinguishes itself from certain key works of fiction about health and racial prejudice from later in the twentieth century that take a more oppositional and antagonistic approach to medical authority. Ann Folwell Stanford has shown how contemporary writers dedicated to racial justice in medicine often have outright rejected conventional biomedical models and instead have privileged other modes of healing and care. In this body of contemporary fiction, including that of Octavia Butler, "the terms of hegemony are reversed as medicine is closed out of the diagnostic and healing process." "Resisting traditional medicine," Folwell Stanford notes, these fictional texts "avoid categories or labels that function as mechanisms of power and strategies of control."[137] Similarly, Martha Cutter shows how forms of informal and collective care in Toni Morrison's fiction can "elide the medical establishment to embody a metacultural ethics of healing."[138] Writing at an earlier moment in which professional medicine's cultural authority was at its peak, the authors discussed in this chapter—Chesnutt, White, and Ellison—focused on trained physicians, nurses, and specialized disciplines such as psychiatry and how they could be reformed and recalibrated to better serve Black patients. In so doing, they pointed to social problems that later writers would continue to critique while offering glimpses of possibilities for solutions that would be administered through medical institutions themselves.

In order to intervene against prejudice's sickening and injurious effects, they anchored scenes of official, institutional medicine to the energies of the racial protest movements sweeping through US society. In so doing, they extended beyond an emphasis on professional representation alone. Their novels not only portrayed individual Black physicians—William in *Marrow*, Ken in *Fire in the Flint*, and the vet in *Invisible Man*—but they insisted on revising the structures, systems, and forms of knowledge integral to modern medical care more broadly. While Chesnutt explored the complications of assimilation and professional advancement within a segregated medical system, he privileged William's hospital as a space of communal empowerment. For White, empowerment could similarly be achieved through channeling a "fighting spirit" against racial violence through the practice of professional medicine, even though the obstacles to professional success were manifold. Ellison, writing later in the twentieth century, called attention to medical harm while also celebrating and advancing reforms to psychiatry. Resisting melodramas of care and unsettling expectations for simplistic forms of compassion within a segregated and unequal medical system, these writers paired a sense of the power of Black medical expertise and knowledge with commitments to reform and radical social change. They gestured toward the ways that medical professionalism, however clinical or dispassionate it might be, could not be politically neutral.

CHAPTER THREE

Sexual Health and Women's Rights

IN *HELEN BRENT, M.D.* (1892)—a novel whose author, Annie Nathan Meyer, "handled with great frankness the theme of social evil"—[1]the titular character encounters a young patient who "timidly" enters the office.[1] It is implied that the visitor suffers from venereal disease,[2] as Brent remarks, "the old, old story."[3] In this scene, both doctor and patient hesitate to mention the disease explicitly. Throughout the novel, Meyer never names venereal disease directly, thereby mirroring the late nineteenth-century culture of secrecy. However, the novel not only portrays this silence but also implicitly critiques it, breaking taboos regarding sexuality, disease, and desire. By depicting characters forced to remain silent about their affliction while enduring pain and suffering, Meyer gestures toward the detrimental effects of a culture of silence and fear on women's health. Meyer held that her book had been "ahead of its day" but that "one critic declared its place was in a doctor's office or laboratory, not in the library of a lay person."[4] In fact, the novel contained within its pages a medical thesis about women's health, but it presented its argument through evocative and suggestive literary prose.

Similar to *Helen Brent, M.D.*, James Oppenheim's *Wild Oats* (1910) is a romantic novel that also functions as sexual health education, attempting to thwart the ravages of venereal disease on women's well-being. In *Wild Oats*, a character named Edith is warned by her mother that there exists a "double-standard, under which men freely go with women before marriage, and girls remain innocent."[5] Initially, Edith believes it is "better to remain ignorant and happy."[6] However, as Edith gradually becomes aware of the realities of venereal disease, Oppenheim instructs his readers that facts about venereal disease can radically—and painfully—alter one's worldview: "Facts are aggressive. They leap at us, sting us, batter a breach, drive into the mind, tear old beliefs to tatters . . ."[7] A central aim of the novel is to compel readers to confront these hard truths, however disquieting. In particular, *Wild Oats* promotes the control of disease by urging men to adjust their matrimonial plans in order to safeguard women's health. Edith insists that her fiancé undergo testing for venereal disease before marriage. In a recurring trope within fiction about sexual health, Frank—who had sown his "wild oats" and become ill from a "woman out West"—learns from his doctor that, despite a claim by "some old chap" that he was "cured for life,"[8] he was never truly cured and might require months or even a year for treatment. Consequently, Frank is advised against marrying until fully treated. The doctor challenges Frank's masculinity in order to prod him to wait: "The world isn't a stage and all the men and women merely players ... And only a real man can grapple with this real life. Are you a real man, Frank?"[9] Here, an ostensibly courageous yet responsible conception of masculinity—one that acknowledges the risks of venereal disease—is encouraged with the aim of preserving women's health. Nevertheless, Frank marries Edith, and their child is born blind as a consequence of the illness. Subsequently, though, the doctor counsels Edith to forgive her husband for transmitting the disease, advice to which she eventually acquiesces. "Now, indeed," the doctor proclaims, "You are truly married."[10] The novel concludes by linking the success of a "real" marriage with the narrative resolution of the venereal disease plot, insisting on men's sexual control even as it allows for forgiveness for breaches of it. Though with different emphases, Meyer and Oppenheim pointed to the social influences impacting the spread of venereal disease and sought to promote women's rights to autonomy and health.

In writing this fiction that promoted women's sexual health, Meyer and Oppenheim were each doing significant cultural and political work, as the official, mainstream response to venereal disease was inflected by deeply repressive and patriarchal attitudes. There was a strong sense that venereal disease should not be talked about, which reformers pointed to as a "conspiracy of silence." This unfolded in the period of the enforcement of the Comstock Laws beginning in 1873. Spearheaded by anti-vice crusader and US postal inspector Anthony Comstock, the Act for the Suppression of Trade in, and Circulation of, Obscene Literature and Articles of Immoral Use, made it illegal to distribute any material deemed "obscene" or "indecent" by US mail, including information on prevention methods for venereal disease.[11] Initially confined to censorship within the US Postal Service, these restrictions eventually extended to private carriers as well. Venereal disease was increasingly becoming policed more broadly. In the early twentieth century, this would eventually culminate in the American Plan, whereby thousands of women were invasively examined for venereal diseases. While the American Plan was initiated during World War I to prevent soldiers and sailors from contracting venereal diseases from "prostitutes," it quickly expanded to include women seen as overly flirtatious or even those who were seen alone in public spaces, and many of those thought to be infected were sent to jails, beaten, and forcibly sterilized.[12]

These patriarchal attitudes toward venereal disease did not go without being critiqued. Prominent New York City venereologist and founder of the Society of Moral Prophylaxis, Prince A. Morrow claimed that venereal disease posed a serious threat to the "relations between the sexes" by negatively impacting women's health: "the conditions created by the marriage relation render the wife a helpless and unresisting victim." In this view, marriage was potentially perilous not only because of the confining strictures of domesticity in general but also because it often deprived women of critical medical knowledge. As Morrow explained, "The *vinculum matrimonii* is a chain which binds and fetters the woman completely, making her the passive recipient of the germs of any sexual disease her husband may harbor. On her wedding night she may, and often does, receive unsuspectingly the poison of a disease which may seriously affect her health and kill her children...."[13] Moreover, Morrow noted that literary texts often reinforced this perspective: "Young women should know that marriage is not all romance and sentiment, that dissipated men make unsafe husbands and unsound fathers," he warned, "and that the halo of romantic interest thrown around the man with a profligate past by fiction writers is a symbol of shame, a signal of danger for his wife and children."[14]

While some authors contributed to the romanticization of men with "profligate" pasts, others rejected this portrayal and instead, as Morrow did, likened oppressive marital conventions to a "chain" that threatened women's health. In particular, Charlotte Perkins Gilman and Upton Sinclair, whom this chapter focuses on, are notable for their extensive engagement with medical conversations and debates about this issue. They crafted narratives that explicitly pointed to solutions to the problems that writers like Meyer and Oppenheim evoked. They attempted to suggest that methods of medical prevention for venereal disease did not have to stifle or constrain women's emotional and sexual lives in order to be effective. Rather, progress could be achieved by crafting new narratives about venereal disease that portrayed women as actively reclaiming control over their health from dangerous, disease-bearing men. As Stephanie Peebles Tavera demonstrates, writers of medical fiction advancing women's rights harped on readers' fears by combining emotional mobilization with scientific expertise to reframe cultural narratives and stereotypes regarding disease transmission.[15] They criticized forms of sexual moralism that were predicated on encouraging compulsory domesticity and instituting double standards of sexual morality: while men were free to sow their "wild oats" before marriage—thereby endangering women's health—middle-class women were advised by doctors to abstain from premarital sex to protect the health of their future husbands and families. In response, these authors championed women's rights to protect themselves within and beyond marriage, advocating for the refusal or dissolution of unions that endangered their sexual health. Both writers relayed what Gilman called the "painful facts"[16] of venereal disease, which they understood as being linked not only to physical symptoms but to deeply psychological concerns. In this light, they combined an emphasis on empiricism and didacticism with a sensitivity to emotional trauma, as expressed through tense, conflict-ridden plots of love and seduction. In their view, effective sexual health education required the strategic mobilization of medical expertise, aligning scientific knowledge with emotional truths to protect women's bodies and minds. They expressed their ideas in their reform work, journalism, and fiction, through which they detailed specific resolutions to various threats posed to women's health. Throughout, they rejected the notion that syphilis and gonorrhea were solely the consequences of prostitution or the result of middle-class women's increasing marital and sexual autonomy in the era of the "New Woman," as many physicians and commentators suggested. Instead, they critiqued the violence, deception, and oppression inflicted on women by men carrying the disease and by a largely patriarchal medical profession. In doing so, they tried to demonstrate how medical knowledge about venereal disease could empower women, as they subverted the moralizing and punitive logics of conventional medicine and masculinist narratives of love to establish women's rights to bodily and psychological autonomy as a critical aim of public health.

At the same time, their writing was influenced by eugenics and forms of state-sanctioned marital regulation that compromised the integrity of their agendas, extending the right to health primarily to white, middle-class, able-bodied women. While these writers mounted critiques of venereal disease treatments that challenged patriarchal medical attitudes, they also presented a troubling, instrumentalized view of women's sexuality that affirmed the kinds of patriarchal authority that, on one level, they sought to challenge. Because venereal disease was not only transmissible between husbands and wives but could also be inherited by children, venereal disease debates came to implicate not only questions of wives' sexual health but also the health of future generations. This era was one in which eugenics – the "science" of reproduction pioneered by Francis Galton that aimed to increase the prevalence of traits perceived to be desirable within the population through mechanisms ranging from marital advice to sterilization – became increasingly popularized. Gilman and Sinclair tethered the aim of protecting women's health to a reproductive future predicated on sexual regulation, revealing a politics of health that was both liberatory and constraining, empowering and compromised.

Courtship, Marriage, and Disease

Shortly following its publication, Charlotte Perkins Gilman remarked on the 1914 medical pamphlet *Never-Told Tales* by New York physician William J. Robinson, noting that "Dr. Robinson is not a novelist by profession," yet "his heart is so wrung and his brain so roused by the hidden tragedy he sees all about him that he has reached out into literature for aid."[17] In this pamphlet, Robinson recounts the story of a marriage destroyed by venereal disease, employing a prose style reminiscent of fiction. Although *Never-Told Tales* was a medical pamphlet, its evocative prose, as Gilman noted, imbued it with a novelistic quality. The relationship between Edward and Rose is rendered with psychological detail and emotional depth. As he describes it, "... Edward—dear Ed, whom she had loved and looked up to for so many years—had proposed last night, and the passion, romance and aroma of that proposal still lingered with her."[18] But after Rose acquires gonorrhea from him and undergoes successful surgery, Robinson observed, "you would hardly know her if you saw her. She aged ten years in ten weeks. She is making no plans, she has no hopes, she is dreaming no dreams—not for the present at any rate. Never again will she be the happy Rose that she was before she became Mrs. Edward. Never will her home be gladdened by the noise, romp and laughter of little children."[19] *Never-Told Tales* addressed not only venereal disease but also divorce, domestic violence, and suicide. Robinson contended that these tragic scenes stemmed from flawed social norms surrounding sexual health rather than from individual failings. He recognized that these issues carried particularly high stakes for women—who were often publicly cast as morally deficient even as their own health was compromised by men.

For Gilman, as for Robinson, controlling venereal disease necessitated a combination of medical and literary tactics. Early scholarly attention to her work—beginning in the 1970s—focused primarily on her resistance to Silas Weir Mitchell's "rest cure," as notably portrayed in her story "The Yellow Wall-Paper" (1892). But Gilman was also engaged in broader debates with doctors about the public health crisis of venereal disease, which was a matter in which women's autonomy and health were both also at stake. For Gilman, this mission required, specifically, blending scientific empiricism with the emotive appeals of fictional love plots—engaging, as per her review of Robinson's work, both the "brain" and the "heart"—to underscore the unique risks that venereal disease posed to women's lives. While Robinson's pamphlet presented a tragedy-infused narrative in which women are depicted as passive victims of a patriarchal society, Gilman advocated for women's sexual health by portraying women as active agents with the power to resist the violence of a medical establishment that had been primarily dominated by men.

Gilman's perspectives on venereal disease were informed by her broader efforts to offer a rational approach to domestic affairs through public health initiatives. She argued that domestic labor should be professionalized and regulated. A generation earlier, domestic advice manuals—such as Gilman's great-aunt Catherine Beecher's *A Treatise on Domestic Economy* (1841)—sought to improve home life by applying scientific principles to housekeeping.[20] Similarly, Gilman aimed to radically transform domesticity to contribute to public health. In her essay "Kitchen-Mindedness" (1910), she asserted that "health is a public concern" and that the "feeding of our people is one of the most vital factors in their health, and that the private kitchen with its private cook is not able to keep the public well." She further urged, "Ask the physician, the sanitary expert, in fighting the filth diseases we have the public forces to work with; compulsory systems of sewage and drainage, quarantine, isolation hospitals, and all the other maneuvers by which an enlightened public protects itself. But who shall say what a child shall eat, or a man or woman? Is it not wholly their own affair?" She critiqued the "narrowness of vision" and "petty self-interest" that would make it so. According to Gilman, only by professionalizing the domestic sphere could the "primitive little shop" of the traditional kitchen be replaced by a "cool glittering laboratory, wherein the needs of bodily replenishment are fully and beautifully met."[21] Unlike the individualized approach of domestic science, Gilman's view of modern public health entailed reframing hitherto private matters as being public concerns through new infrastructures and expert medical oversight.

This shift toward public health in domestic affairs carried significant implications for women's health in general and their sexual health in particular. In *Women and Economics* (1898), Gilman argued that women suffered due to their economic dependence on men and attributed the pervasive "horror" of disease to a "pathological maternity."[22] To remedy this, she advocated for women's involvement in regimented and scientific domestic systems. Gilman criticized the reliance on conventional "public means" for not going far enough. This included sanitary regulations, medical inspections, social hygiene literature, and "special legislation" targeting "contagious diseases and dangerous trades" (a reference to prostitution and the spread of venereal disease). Gilman observed that too often "the health that lies in the hands of the housewife is not reached by these measures."[23] Gilman's discussion of venereal disease underscored her belief that public health must emerge through domestic routes as well, and she noted the particular need to protect middle-class women from venereal disease. In *The Forerunner*, Gilman wrote, "The spread of social ethics among the medical profession is cause for great rejoicing." Enthralled by advances in "social sanitation," she applauded governmental efforts at both local and national levels to protect US citizens from venereal disease.[24]

Nevertheless, Gilman was critical of pervasive secrecy surrounding sexual health issues. Even as authorities policed venereal diseases, there remained a reluctance to discuss them openly. To counter this culture of secrecy, Gilman frequently compared venereal diseases to other contagious diseases in an effort to lessen the stigma surrounding them. For example, in the same *Forerunner* article in which she reviewed Robinson's work, Gilman observed, "If the doctors come forward to tell us how the typhoid bacillus is disseminated and how dangerous it is, and how it is to be avoided, we are interested, grateful and more or less willing to profit by the instruction. But when they try to tell us how the gonococcus attacks humanity, how dangerous it is, and how it is to be avoided, we say 'Sh! That is something you musn't talk about!'"[25] Accordingly, Gilman demanded that doctors register cases of venereal disease just as they did for other contagious diseases.

Gilman's writings reveal both the progressive and deeply troubling dimensions of her views on sexual health. Although her ideas about marriage, motherhood, and chastity were rooted in nineteenth-century maternalism, she adapted these concepts into a modern argument for women's sexual health. Troublingly, Gilman was also a eugenicist—invested in preserving whiteness and able-bodied identities against perceived threats of national "degeneration" through sexual regulation and discipline. She was not alone in this regard; eugenics became deeply intertwined with Progressive Era discourse on sexual health. For example, public health reformer and nurse Lavinia Dock asserted that "the education of fathers and mothers, must, in the future, include the principles of heredity, the toxic effect of unholy passions upon temperament and character, and the study of eugenics, the new science for the improvement of the race of man."[26] Similarly, Prince Albert Morrow argued in *Social Diseases and Marriage* (1904) for women's sexual health in terms that were connected to his fears about the "degeneration of the race."[27] Such arguments were predicated on biological essentialism; Morrow contended that venereal diseases threatened the "instinct of maternity"—a trait he saw as "implanted by nature in every normally constituted woman" as "her highest destiny in being created a woman."[28] As was the case for Dock and Morrow, despite Gilman's intentions to contribute to women's liberation, her eugenic rhetoric conferred scientific authority to already-entrenched, troubling patriarchal attitudes toward sex and reproduction. Her emphasis on public health as a women's rights issue marked an attempt to craft a progressive politics of care, but it turned out to be deeply flawed. That Gilman's attempt at securing women's rights to sexual health was troublingly exclusionary can be seen in *Concerning Children* (1903), in which she asserted that "if a young man and woman are clean, healthy, vigorous, and virtuous before parenthood, they may become dirty, sickly, weak, and wicked afterward with far less ill effect to the race than if they were sick and vicious before their children were born, and thereafter became stalwart saints. The sowing of wild oats would be far less harmful if sowed in the autumn instead of in the spring." Through couching her ideas in euphemism and seasonal metaphors, Gilman articulated a harmful eugenic agenda. While early scholarship on Gilman celebrated her advocacy for women's agency and health, later critics have focused on her complicity in this kind of eugenic ideology. As this later wave of scholarship has shown, in privileging a naturalized sense of women's reproductive roles and biological motherhood, Gilman sought to serve the interests of only some (white, middle-class) American women,[29] and to forestall notions of degeneration and "race suicide." In so doing, Gilman also inevitably presented an instrumentalized view of women's sexuality. As Linda Gordon observes, eugenic ideology is deeply restrictive, as it presupposes that "reproduction was not just a function but the purpose, in some teleological sense, of a woman's life."[30] Mary Ziegler similarly notes that eugenic feminism was based on the idea that "women must be granted more reproductive freedom," but it was achieved through a "movement that called for more regulation of female sexual behavior and reproduction."[31] It is critical to distinguish between the task of protecting women's health and eugenic ideologies, but Gilman conflated them. While she was dedicated to protecting women's health, her commitment to the state-sanctioned disciplining and surveillance of courtship and marriage to stave off perceived threats of degeneration compromised her mission.

In her reform work, Gilman endeavored to reconcile an inherently misogynist eugenic ideology with a public health agenda aimed at empowering women, which meant that her mission was inherently paradoxical. In a 1910 speech to the Society of Moral Prophylaxis, she framed sexual health education as crucial to addressing issues that disproportionately affected women, asserting that venereal disease is "infinitely more wicked in its effects on the wife and child" than on the husband. She advocated for more open discussions of sexual health, arguing, ". . . if you are compelled to tell that a man has leprosy, or cholera, or the plague, that breaks the Hippocratic oath into so many pieces that it cannot be restored. There is no reason why it should apply to these diseases and not to others." In advocating for such protections, Gilman contended that venereal disease "robs the mother of the power to fulfill her functional duty," a statement that revealed her view that healthy maternalism was not only a right (a "power") but also a social responsibility (a "duty").[32]

The Crux (1911) contains Gilman's most extensive elaborations on women's rights to transparent information about sexual health, even as the novel is paradoxically governed by a regressive eugenic ideology. The narrative centers on a Colorado community organized around a boarding house called "The Cottonwoods." Run by Dr. Jane Bellair, the boarding house becomes a refuge for the protagonist, Vivian Lane, whom Jane brings from her New England home. Jane advises Vivian against marrying Morton Elder, a man afflicted with syphilis. Jane became a doctor expressly to "save other women" from disease after forsaking marriage to a man who carried gonorrhea—a circumstance that had prevented her from bearing healthy children.[33] Consistent with the politics of social motherhood pervasive in Gilman's work, Jane treats Vivian as a surrogate daughter, remarking, "If she had had a daughter, perhaps she would have been like that. If she had had a daughter, would she not have thanked anyone who would try to save her from such a danger? From that worse than deadly peril, because of which she had no daughter."[34] In a strategic appeal to what she perceives to be Vivian's maternal instincts, Jane warns, "Think about their lovely little soft helplessness—when you hold them . . ."[35] Jane contends that if Vivian were to marry Morton, her children would be at risk of becoming "crippled," "idiots," "blind," and might die prematurely.[36] The full implications of this eugenic ideology are further revealed by Vivian's grandmother, Mrs. Pettigrew, who informs Vivian that women's clubs and congresses "have become more aware of venereal diseases, leading to some states passing laws requiring a medical certificate—a clean bill of health—to go with a license to marry."[37] In staging these parallel views, Gilman portrays a disciplinary regime of public health that extends from the doctor's counsel into the very fabric of domestic life.

Gilman's portrayal of Jane —who directs maternalist care toward the community—entailed imagining a politics of collective health beyond the restrictive confines of the nuclear family. As Cynthia Davis explains, Gilman consistently avoided overemphasizing what she referred to as the "extended self" of the individual family.[38] In depicting Jane's displaced domestic motivations for her medical practice, Gilman tried to resolve some of the longstanding tensions between domesticity and social responsibility that had troubled her. Reflecting on her own conflicted desires about marriage in her autobiography, Gilman recalled, "My mind was not fully clear as to whether I should or should not marry. On the one hand I knew it was normal and right in general, and held that a woman should be able to have marriage and motherhood, and do her work in the world also. On the other, I felt strongly that for me it was not right, that the nature of the life before me forbade it, that I ought to forego the more intimate personal happiness for complete devotion to my work." After marrying Walter Stetson,

Gilman suffered from depression and anxiety; eventually, she divorced him and dedicated herself to work, public service, lecturing, and reform efforts—though she remained anxious about the competing imperatives of marriage versus her professional and social obligations.[39] This kind of conflict between domesticity and broader social engagement is resolved in *The Crux* through images of sentimental, quasi-familial bonds taking shape through the practice of medicine—a field she regarded as having the potential to advance women's health. Cindy Weinstein observes that "sentimental fictions delineate alternative models of sympathy which, when examined, enrich our understanding of the multiple ways in which sympathy was imagined and practiced." Weinstein critiques the view that sentimental fiction exclusively privileges the biological family, noting that many American novels "tell the surprisingly pragmatic stories of these other 'parents' and their ability or lack thereof to have sympathy for children who are not, biologically speaking, theirs" and, consequently, "to extend the meaning of family is to extend the possibilities for sympathy."[40] Throughout *The Crux*, Gilman broadens the scope of sympathetic attachment by portraying a flexible form of care that permeates diverse social relations—extending beyond familial bonds to the doctor–patient relationship.

Through the portrayal of Jane's medical advice and the way it shapes Vivian's decisions, Gilman challenges medical secrecy. As Martha Cutter notes, the "free circulation of medical discourse" was paramount to Gilman. US doctors argued that disclosing a patient's sexual health status to their partner would violate Hippocratic principles and lead to stigmatization. Physicians feared that such revelations might precipitate marital dissolution and drive patients away from mainstream medicine toward quackery.[41] Nevertheless, some physicians, while generally upholding patient confidentiality, contended that exceptions should be made in certain cases of venereal disease. For example, Prince Albert Morrow argued that "while the obligation of the medical secret is in the general interest of the social order, and should be maintained as a fixed principle of professional conduct, it may be admitted that a situation of a peculiarly aggravating character may present itself when the patient shows himself an exceptional sort of brute by the obstinacy with which he adheres to his criminal purposes after he is assured that he will almost certainly infect his wife . . ." In such cases, Morrow maintained, exceptions to confidentiality were justified.[42] In advocating for similar breaches of patient confidentiality to protect women's health, Gilman intervened in contemporary debates over medical ethics. Notably, before Jane discloses Morton's disease to Vivian, she attempts to persuade Dick Hale—Morton's physician—to disclose the relevant details of his patient's condition. This scene foregrounds the complex relationship between medical professionalism, ethics, and the politics of compassion. In the ensuing debate over patient confidentiality, Dick dismisses Jane's reimagined maternal responsibility toward Vivian as unprofessional: "I am not Miss Lane's father, brother, uncle or guardian . . ."[43] He notes, "It's a matter of honor—professional honor. You women don't seem to know what the word means,"[44] Jane retorts, "You don't have to kill Vivian Lane . . . A man's honor always seems to want to kill a woman to satisfy it. I'm glad I haven't got the feeling."[45] According to Dick, professionalism demands dispassion; he privileges the strict adherence to confidentiality over Vivian's health—even her life. By asserting that he is not related to Vivian, he rejects any sentimentality. Yet when Jane contends that Dick's sense of honor is merely a "feeling," she undermines the notion that professionalism can be neutral. Within a patriarchal medical establishment, Dick's brand of professionalism ultimately endangers women's health—a notion encapsulated by the comment about patient confidentiality "killing" Vivian. In contrast, professional medical women like Jane have cultivated what Gilman views as the proper kind of feeling, strategically channeled toward protecting women's health and lives.

Jane's advice to Vivian to reject Morton is intended to protect Vivian's right to health as a key aspect of her autonomy, but it is inflected by Gilman's eugenic mission. Gilman was not unique in framing informed consent as a public health issue nor in doing so in a manner that was, unfortunately, influenced by eugenic ideology. Early articulations of this perspective, pairing health, consent, and fears of "degeneration" emerged in the oratory of suffrage leader and free-love reformer Victoria Woodhull. In an 1873 address, Woodhull denounced "enforced intercourse as in marriage" for "sending thousands of wives" "annually . . . to untimely graves" but also for producing a "world peopled by intellectual, moral, or social dwarfs and abortions;" [46] she questioned whether "children begotten under the rule of love and consent . . . can possibly be bad?"[47] For birth-control reformer Margaret Sanger, in the early twentieth century, sexual choice was not only a right but also a social responsibility; in *Woman and the New Race* (1920), the title of which reveals its eugenic leanings, she argued that "woman was and is condemned to a system under which the lawful rapes exceed the unlawful ones a million to one. She has nothing to say as to whether she shall have strength sufficient to give a child a fair physical and mental start in life."[48] Similarly, in the sexual health advice book *The Three Gifts of Life* (1913), Nellie May Smith—a lecturer for the Society of Sanitary and Moral Prophylaxis—contended that young women "speak of falling in love as if it were something over which they have no control; but they can control it in a certain way,"[49] and she warned that men might drug women to place them "completely under [their] control," cautioning against allowing men to "take any liberty" with them.[50] Yet Smith's arguments for sexual autonomy and consent were articulated within a eugenic logic aimed at advancing "race progress": according to her, young women seeking "strong, healthy children" should marry "strong and clean and healthy" husbands to secure a "good inheritance" for their offspring.[51] For many reformers, sexual autonomy and public health went hand in hand, but troublingly, these were in turn interconnected with eugenic ideology. *The Crux* resonates with these broader currents of reform and brings them to bear on the treatment of venereal disease, which plays out through Vivian's resistance to her suitor Morton's violence, enabled by Jane's eugenically tinged advice. Prior to Jane's warning, Vivian is deeply ambivalent about Morton. In their first encounter, he makes unwanted sexual advances, and Vivian hesitates before his kiss—though she finds it difficult to articulate her discomfort: "It is difficult—it is well nigh impossible—for a girl to put a name to certain small cuddlings not in themselves terrifying, nor even unpleasant, but which she obscurely feels to be wrong."[52] After he kisses her goodbye, she struggles to "arrange in her mind this mixture of grief, disapproval, shame and triumph" that the kiss has evoked.[53] Later, at a social dance in the West, when Morton forcefully presses on her, Vivian deliberately turns away, and she "tried to withdraw herself, but he held her fast." Eventually, Morton coerces Vivian into agreeing to marry him; as he grips her, she pleads, "You hurt me!" and he replies, "Say yes, dear, and I'll let you go—for a little while." Only after this promise of only partial release does Vivian say, under pressure, "yes."[54] These moments of coercion and violence illustrate that Vivian's refusals of Morton are assertions of her sexual autonomy. In rendering these details, Gilman positions intimacy not only as a personal matter but as a public health issue. By foregrounding Jane's counsel against Morton's aggressive advances, Gilman makes autonomy and consent central to her vision of sexual health. At the same time, troublingly, like other progressive public health reformers, Gilman does so in *The Crux* while binding consent and public health to a eugenic mission.

After Vivian's rejection of Morton, Gilman reinforces her argument that socially maternalist care serves as an antidote to sexual violence and risky marriages. Vivian embraces social motherhood by working in childcare at a kindergarten, where she teaches children (especially young women) "physical culture," thereby contributing to the novel's didactic aim of educating youth about health risks.[55] As she cares for the children, whatever remains of her lovesickness for Morton dissipates in the face of "the loving touch of little hands, the gay contentment of her well-ordered charges."[56] This moment echoes Jane's earlier remarks about the joy of holding "tender infants" which she had noted Vivian would forgo if she married Morton. Crucially, the kind of maternalist care that Vivian now engages in extends beyond marriage and biological motherhood, as she educates other parents' children about public health.

An expansive sense of care, which fosters safety and security, promises protection against seduction, patriarchal violence, and even the inherent risks of marriage. Morton's first kiss with Vivian had been portrayed as horrifying and is later identified by Jane as a threat to Vivian's health. While Vivian's friend Adela praises the "sweetness" of a typical first kiss, encouraging her to embrace Morton's advances, Vivian reacts with visible discomfort—rising abruptly and moving toward the window. Then Vivian kisses Adela. Here, Gilman subtly implies such a friendship might pose an alternative to, and supplant the kind of violence enacted by, Morton's sexual aggression.[57] Notably, in the novel's concluding lines, Adela herself laments that her return to the east will "end so many pleasant friendships,"[58] as Gilman hints at the valorization of platonic friendships and care between women as forms of intimacy that might be free from both conflict and disease.

Yet between the representation of this romantic friendship and these concluding lines that privilege that kind of friendship once again, for Gilman there still has to be a marriage. Since the novel ends with Vivian marrying Dick, Gilman appears to ultimately align her vision of a national reproductive future with patriarchal medical authority, which is the very authority she initially critiques. Crucially, however, Dick has been reformed by the novel's end. Whereas Morton is rendered an untenable husband for Vivian—having sown his "wild oats"[59]—Dick demonstrates self-control. His initial prioritization of professionalism over his desire to marry Vivian proves his capacity to regulate his sexual urges in the interests of public health. Gilman asserts that medical wisdom must rein in passionate, impulsive desires, while interpersonal ethics and a sense of social responsibility must prevail over unthinking sexual fulfillment. Dick possesses both medical knowledge and the awareness of the risks inherent in romantic desire. By disavowing his misogyny, he becomes, in Gilman's rendering, a suitable husband. In a way, Dick's capacity for transformation through marriage parallels Vivian's own change of course following Jane's medical counsel. Just as medical women work to reform the institution of marriage in order to protect sexual health, the ostensibly right kind of marriage—predicated on consent and autonomy, but also troublingly, shaped by eugenic ideology—ultimately reforms the patriarchal doctor.

Gilman's critique of attitudes toward venereal disease expressed in *The Crux* is further evident in her short story "Wild Oats and Tame Wheat" (1913). In the story, a man has "sowed his wild oats"—that is, he has "loved—or what he called love—freely"—and we learn that "among other acquisitions he acquired one or two diseases not easily dismissed, so he perforce retained them." Gilman's euphemistic language describing his acquisition of "diseases" both registers and critiques the culture of secrecy surrounding venereal diseases. This coded language continues in the depiction of the "damsel" he marries, who has "sowed no wild oats, but much tame wheat." Upon their marriage, it is revealed that "she knew little, even of the life of him she lived with, though he shared with her what he thought fit, including his diseases."[60] Though employing a light tone, Gilman posed a serious challenge to the double standard of sexual morality that pervaded both men's expectations and women's attitudes regarding venereal disease. "Wild Oats and Tame Wheat" underscores the necessity of transparency by reducing information asymmetries about venereal disease as well as promoting the regulation of men's sexual activities.

Although Gilman advocated for the restraint of men's sexual urges to protect public health, she often framed venereal disease as a social problem rather than an individual moral failing. In her short story "The Vintage" (1916), Gilman introduces Leslie, from a "good family" in the South who is "proud of her blazing health."[61] After falling in love with both a young doctor, Faulkner, and a college classmate, Moore, Leslie ultimately chooses to marry Moore. Prior to the wedding, Moore discovers a throat infection, and Faulkner informs him that he has acquired syphilis and was never properly cured. Through this story, Gilman critiques a culture of secrecy and shame surrounding venereal disease. Although Faulkner appears well-intentioned, his strict adherence to patient confidentiality jeopardizes Leslie's health: "What else could he do? He was a physician with a high sense of professional honor. The physician must not betray his patient."[62] As opposed to *The Crux*, in which Morton is presented as explicitly aggressive, the lack of open communication regarding sexual health renders the men in "The Vintage" as unwitting vehicles of entrenched patriarchal views. When Moore consults Faulkner, Faulkner advises him to undergo testing for venereal disease, but Moore refuses. The narrator explains, "Understand—he did not really in cold blood decide to offer such a risk to the woman he loved. He refused to admit that there was a risk."[63] Rather than being presented as villainous, Moore is an unwitting participant in a culture of secrecy who does not fully realize the harm he causes.

After Moore proceeds with his marriage to Leslie despite Faulkner's medical counsel, he watches Leslie's health deteriorate before she dies, and when their child learns that it was venereal disease that caused his mother's death, he sympathetically exclaims, "Oh my poor father!"[64] For Gilman, it is crucial that both the child's and the readers' sympathy extend even to the father who inadvertently introduced venereal disease into the family. The unfolding tragedy is presented not solely as Moore's fault but as the inevitable result of inadequate sexual health education, which negatively affects wives, husbands, and children.

Gilman would continue to remain active in sexual health reform alongside *The Crux* and her short fiction about venereal disease. The contours of her sexual health agenda appeared again in her response to physician Hugh Cabot's 1916 remarks in Washington, DC, which criticized the mandatory reporting of venereal disease. Beginning with an 1899 Michigan law, many states had enacted marriage laws aimed at eliminating venereal disease from families by requiring medical examinations and certificates attesting that prospective husbands were disease-free.[65] At the Congress of American Physicians and Surgeons, Cabot noted that by that time, eleven states (California, Connecticut, Indiana, Iowa, Kansas, Louisiana, Michigan, Ohio, Utah, Vermont, and Wisconsin) had mandated that physicians report venereal diseases such as syphilis to public health authorities.[66] He argued that controlling venereal disease should depend on individuals acting in socially responsible ways rather than on formal, restrictive legislation—which he contended would engender a "false sense of security."[67] Instead of such legislation, he recommended that states, cities, and hospitals invest more extensively in the diagnosis, treatment, and supervision of venereal disease.

After encountering Hugh Cabot's address in the journal of the American Social Hygiene Association, Gilman expressed agreement with his view that US society needed to better control venereal disease. However, she criticized his refusal to endorse mandatory reporting. For Gilman, Cabot's emphasis on guarding individual liberty from government interference was overly general and failed to account for the concrete particularities of women's health. While she concurred with his assertion that "if Society should fail to control syphilis, syphilis would control Society,"[68] she found his opposition to reporting these cases troubling given the potential threat that this posed to women's health. Cabot dismissed critics who contended that women's suffrage would automatically resolve the venereal disease crisis. In contrast, Gilman and others advocated for pragmatic measures—such as monitoring men's sexual health—to address the double standard of sexual morality. Noting that there were very few documented cases of women infecting grooms, she maintained that laws regulating disease transmission were necessary: Gilman wrote that "for a man to voluntarily inoculate an innocent loving wife and even the unborn child with a hideous disease is a plain crime and should be so treated, so punished."[69]

Gilman's advocacy for sexual health involved urging the restraint of men's sexual activity. She argued that men should be ashamed of behaviors that facilitated the spread of venereal disease and instead she placed a premium on monogamy. For example, consider her response to a 1914 debate between physicians Richard Cabot and William J. Robinson regarding sexual health. While these physicians each thought differently about the value of disease prevention, in Gilman's view they both failed to account sufficiently for women's agency and health.

Richard Cabot viewed a modern, disciplinary public health regime as a threat to conventional values of marriage, maternity, and chastity. Speaking to the Society of Sanitary and Moral Prophylaxis—the first US social hygiene association founded by Morrow in New York City—Cabot contended that sanitary measures and morality were fundamentally at odds. He noted that attempts to implement venereal disease prophylaxis in the US Navy resulted in "immoral" behavior by increasing men's sexual contacts. Morality could lead to disease, he acknowledged, but that was sometimes necessary. "I have known women," he remarked, "—you have probably known women—who thought it their duty and their privilege to bear children, even though they knew that childbirth was fraught with danger to health. Morality in that case is bad for sanitation; obeying conscience is in this instance bad for health. But such women take the risk, and I honor them for taking it."[70] For Cabot, any interference of public health regulations in individuals' sexual lives would compromise their morality, which he believed entailed monogamous marriage and maternal duty. While he conceded that public health could be advanced through "spreading facts," "word of mouth," and "reading," he maintained that "the sacredness of motherhood; the responsibilities of parents, the duties of the father, the sanctity of the home, and the sacredness of the human body" were "not within the power of science to teach."[71]

William J. Robinson criticized Richard Cabot's position as absurdly conservative, arguing that since illicit sexual encounters were inevitable, sexual health education and prophylaxis were essential. Regarding men in the US Navy, Robinson advocated for providing "venereal prophylactics" so they could return to their communities without endangering their wives and children.[72] He posited that men's acting upon their sexual desires was "an expression of a perfectly natural instinct" that was not immoral and in fact could not be suppressed, necessitating physical forms of disease prevention.[73]

Despite their differences, both Cabot and Robinson centered their arguments, implicitly, on the rights of men, which Gilman was compelled to critique. Cabot expressed essentialist views about women's roles as wives and mothers and disregarded measures to guard against health risks posed to them, viewing these as inevitable. At the same time, Robinson held that men simply could not control their sexual desires even when their desires put women's health at risk. In fact, his misogynist views became very explicit when he noted regarding Cabot that he "messes things up as badly as any old woman in our Moral Prophylactic Societies," pitting an image of outdated moralism against his own modern scientific authority.[74] In response to the approaches of both Cabot and Robinson, Gilman centered women's health, reiterating the views she had expressed in her fiction. In *The Forerunner*, she lent her support to Robinson's public health policies as opposed to Cabot's criticism of preventative measures , but she critiqued even Robinson's tolerance for men's serial sexual encounters. She maintained that men should not merely indulge their sexual whims, arguing instead that society should prioritize "the woman's capacity for bearing children, not the man's capacity for enjoying himself."[75] For Gilman, public health measures would have to entail challenging conventional forms of venereal disease control and disciplining men's rather than women's sexual lives. Unfortunately, in her intervention in this debate, as was the case throughout much of her work, her ultimate aim was to contribute to a fraught project of national "regeneration" rather than asserting the need to secure women's rights to sexual health and autonomy for their own sake.

Beyond Silence

As Gilman was attempting to critique misogynist US responses to venereal disease, Upton Sinclair closely followed and participated in developments in sexual health reform, including publishing his novel *Sylvia's Marriage* (1914), which he wrote with the inspiration and help of his wife, Mary Craig Sinclair. Sinclair, a major US novelist and reformer, is known for his reform efforts in socialism, temperance, and public health, all of which he conveyed through his muckraking fiction. Criticism of Sinclair's writing on public health has primarily focused on his canonical work *The Jungle* (1905). However, recent scholarship has begun to excavate how Sinclair's corpus—and his unpublished work—engaged with a variety of health-related concerns that extended beyond food safety, including the intersection of sexual health and women's rights.[76]

Shortly after the publication of *The Crux*, Sinclair's novelization of French playwright Eugene Brieux's play *Les Avariés* (1901), entitled *Damaged Goods*, was published in 1913. In it, Sinclair drew inspiration from Brieux's critiques of society's failures to control venereal disease in ways that would protect women's health. When the central character, George DuPont, visits his doctor, he is warned against marrying Henriette while infected with syphilis; the doctor explains that marrying Henriette would entail transmitting the infection to her—and she might even die from it. Nevertheless, George marries Henriette. Subsequently, the novel's characters attempt to assign blame. Henriette's father, Loches, exclaims, "it is the poisoned blood of the prostitute which poisons my daughter and her child; that abject creature, she lives, she lives in us!"[77] He insists, "We must proceed . . . against these miserable women—veritable poisoners that they are!"[78] Ultimately, *Damaged*

Goods endorses the doctor's perspective when he reminds Loches, "You forget that they have first been poisoned. Every one of these women who communicates the disease has first received it from some man."[79] Rather than seeking to punish "prostitutes" for carrying the disease, *Damaged Goods* suggests that men are to blame for transmitting venereal disease to women—whether these women are prostitutes or wives. Moreover, the novel gestures toward the socioeconomic causes of prostitution; the doctor argues that "the prostitute was what she was, not because of innate vileness, but because of economic conditions."[80]

This critique is not without its imperfections. Even as *Damaged Goods* attempts to advance a critique of a patriarchal medical system, it simultaneously reinforces tropes of women's passivity as men debate the best course of action. In addition, Charlotte Perkins Gilman—whose own writing engaged with literary depictions of venereal disease—raised some critiques of her own. She criticized the 1913 theatrical version of *Damaged Goods* arranged by the *Medical Review of Reviews*. She wished that the production had made a more explicit case for protecting women's sexual health. In *The Crux*, Gilman had attempted to blend emotional, personal elements with scientific, factual discourse. While she regarded *Damaged Goods* as "descriptive, informing, moving in the facts presented," she believed it lacked "the personal interest which makes one care for the sufferers." Gilman was also critical that the play offered no solution to the patriarchal threats it exposed: "in the whole discussion of what might be done to check the spread of syphilis and protect the family, no one suggested masculine continence, and no one suggested warning the young women who confront this terrible danger when they marry."[81] Although the theatrical version made some progress, it fell short of advocating for specific reforms in medical practice and public health. Sinclair's novelized version could be critiqued similarly: while women's health is central, the novel features men debating its significance, portraying middle-class women primarily as victims of disease. Moreover, it does not clearly chart a path toward resolving the issues it exposes.

Elsewhere, however, Sinclair proposed specific interventions to promote women's health. Known for his muckraking exposure of social problems, Sinclair had little patience for taboos, moralism, and silence surrounding venereal disease. In a letter to an acquaintance, he emphasized the importance of public health in revising moral standards related to love, marriage, and sex: "I was brought up a Christian," Sinclair wrote, "and I followed the ascetic ideal until I married. I have since come to think that ideal perverted, but on the other hand I have seen so many deplorable results of promiscuous experimenting among radicals that I am very cautious in the ideas I set forth. We are in a transitional stage, and it is very hard to outline a formula that will fit the material facts and the spiritual aspirations. That is hard in other fields than sex. I do not believe in the present institution of marriage-plus-prostitution. I do believe in early marriage, with divorce by mutual consent at any time. All of our thinking about sex must at the present stage of things be conditioned by the fact of venereal disease, which is so wide-spread, so subtle, and difficult to be sure about. On this account any sensible person would wish to keep very close to monogamy..."[82] Sinclair was not advancing a Victorian-era moralistic argument for monogamy but rather promoting a modern sexual health politics that was anchored, much like Gilman's, to the progressivism of his era.

In a 1913 article entitled "Happy Marriage: How Can It Be Assured?" published in *Physical Culture*, Sinclair criticized pervasive secrecy surrounding venereal disease. To do so, he cited examples from Prince A. Morrow's writings, in which he remarked upon physicians deliberately concealing the disease: "the doctor has to treat the husband and deceive the wife, or treat the wife and deceive the husband." Sinclair was particularly concerned with a culture of sexual respectability that adversely affected women. He paid special attention to cases where "the wife has found out the truth, but won't let the husband know that she knows, because if he knew that she knew, she would feel that her self-respect required her to break up the family!"[83] Furthermore, Sinclair noted that the physical symptoms of venereal disease were particularly pronounced for women: "it is especially destructive of the health of women," he claimed, observing that "nearly all the vaginal and uterine infections which make work for the gynecological surgeon are due to it."[84] Sinclair prioritized preserving women's health, and thought appropriate strategies for this were reducing the number of marriages and loosening strictures on divorce. Sinclair described marriage as a potential "trap" and argued that it should be "a good deal easier for people to get divorced, and a good deal harder for them to get married."[85] In particular, he described it as a young man's "first duty" to find a physician, to be medically examined, and to have his physician write to his potential wife with the results. While his potential wife might "tell him out of politeness that he need not do it," he noted she would be "foolish" to "take the chances of an unhappy marriage out of politeness, or kindness of heart, or prudery, or passion, or desire for a home—or for any other reason whatsoever."[86] Later in the article, Sinclair noted that he himself could not reveal as much as he would like, in print, about the prevention of venereal disease because the "Post Office Department" was censoring this kind of information, a reference to the effects of the Comstock laws. If Sinclair thought prudery in young women to be "foolish," he recognized that it was in fact encouraged by American society. Noting the nation was still in the "Dark Ages of Sex-prudery," he remarked that it had "some dark, unventilated dungeons especially provided with tuberculosis germs for the removing of all would-be advocates of sex-reform."[87] Because it contributed to the spread of disease, Sinclair linked a culture of prudery to an illness itself.

Sinclair's response could entail calling for regimented and disciplinary state-sanctioned measures to prevent the spread of venereal disease. As Gilman did, Sinclair called for mandatory reporting of grooms' sexual health status before marriage. He proclaimed: "I will state my reputation as a prophet upon the prediction that if you practice physical culture carefully, and manage to hang onto your life for fifty years more, you will see such marriage laws as the above in force in every State in this Union; and that moreover you will see such a public sentiment on the question that a couple who seek to evade such laws will be regarded as a girl in good society would now be regarded if she were found in a brothel."[88] It is critical to note that for Sinclair, blame for the spread of venereal disease should not rest solely on a "girl in good society" who transgresses marital norms, but on the husband as well. However, Sinclair's ideas about stringent marriage laws regulated by the state marked a repressive dimension of thought.

Resonating with his journalistic writing on the topic, in *Sylvia's Marriage* (1914)—published shortly after *Damaged Goods*—Sinclair's attempts at grounding the discourse of sexual health in women's rights are cast in their fullest relief. As the sequel to *Sylvia*, *Sylvia's Marriage* is narrated by Mary Abbott, a women's rights advocate who divorces her abusive husband before forging an intimate friendship with Sylvia Castleman. The novel begins after Sylvia marries the aristocratic Douglas van Tuiver, and Sylvia and Douglas later have a child, Elaine, who is born blind after Douglas brings gonorrhea into their marriage. At the novel's end, Sylvia even convinces her father to help her sister avoid what she has perceived as her own earlier mistakes by having her sister seek medical advice about a suitor before marriage, at which point the novel becomes affected by fears of "degeneration" and shades of eugenic thought as well.

It is specifically the "medical secret" surrounding venereal disease that enables Douglas to act with impunity, and it is one of Sinclair's primary objects of critique. Dr. Perrin argues that "letting in the light" by informing Sylvia of her illness after her child's birth would only jeopardize her marital relationship—a consequence the doctors deem unacceptable.[89] However, Mary notes that if Sylvia were to be informed of accurate knowledge about venereal disease, she would be better positioned to protect her health. At this point, Mary rejects the notion that Sylvia's relationship would be threatened, and she accuses Perrin of thinking "it was possible to predict what the attitude of any woman be" (219). While it is true that Perrin is overgeneralizing, knowledge of venereal disease does strain Sylvia's relationship, but the novel will in fact endorse her rebellion. Mary notes that Perrin's desire to promote medical secrecy is "based on a peculiar experience he had had—a woman patient who said to him, 'Doctor, I know what is the matter with me, but for God's sake don't let my husband find out that I know, because then I should feel that my self-respect required me to leave him!'"[90] This patient's case echoes one of the scenarios Sinclair pointed to in his 1913 *Physical Culture* article "Happy Marriage," in which a patient's feigned ignorance was a strategy for protecting her marriage. Sinclair suggests this very scenario is tragic, and women should in fact feel emboldened to discuss these matters with their husbands. But in *Sylvia's Marriage*, Sinclair also uses this scene to imply a contrast with the case of Sylvia, who has not been given the opportunity to access accurate information about venereal disease to begin with. In light of layers of secrecy, Sinclair insists that the medical profession must be reformed in a way that privileges transparency, so that husbands and wives could engage in mutual dialogue about these matters rather than keeping them secret.

In fact, Sinclair contends that both the doctors' and Douglas's secrecy is deeply troubling. The doctors' insistence on secrecy is unprofessional. When Mary attempts to persuade Dr. Perrin and his colleague, Dr. Gibson, to prompt Douglas to disclose Sylvia's infection, Gibson retorts that she is "asking us to overstep the bounds of our professional duty. It is not for the physician to decide upon the attitude a wife should take toward her husband."[91] But the very notion of what professional duty entails remains contested. Sinclair suggests that by keeping venereal disease secret, the medical profession is already interfering in their patients' marriages. The doctors view their duty as ensuring Sylvia fulfills her own "duty" to her husband rather than informing her honestly about a condition affecting her own body. But when it comes to these socially and politically charged concerns, medical professionalism cannot remain neutral. Sinclair contrasts the physicians' self-conception with Mary's more enlightened view of what professionalism should entail. Although the doctors claim that their "duty" prohibits meddling in Sylvia and Douglas's marriage, Mary tells Gibson that such an intervention would effectively force Douglas "to accept his opinion of what a wife's duty is."[92] When Perrin later instructs Mary to set aside her "convictions" and consider Sylvia's health—telling Mary that she is the "only person who can calm her" and therefore "surely" it is her "duty to do so"—he conceals the fact that his own strict adherence to a particular conception of professional duty jeopardizes Sylvia's health.[93] In contrast, Mary has a better understanding of medical professionalism. Although Douglas later dismisses her as an "ignorant farmer's wife"[94] for attempting to subvert the authority of the "best physicians in the country," she presses the doctors to acknowledge their obligation to protect Sylvia by providing her with essential medical information. She recognizes that, as with Dick in *The Crux*, the physicians' self-proclaimed professionalism is vulnerable to distortion by patriarchal attitudes.

In contrast, Mary herself comes to assume a kind of medical authority by privileging even the most technical and academic forms of knowledge. Rather than undermining medical expertise, Mary demonstrates her own medical proficiency when she refers to the "virulent gonococcus" that threatens Sylvia and her child—though she remarks it has a "long name."[95] In fact, Mary fully embraces modern medical notions about venereal disease, noting that Perrin remained unaware of these ideas because of his subpar training at an ill-equipped Southern medical college. The point is not that professional medical expertise is unimportant, but that notions of what constitutes such expertise are relative and often inflected by misogynistic bias. Facing these limitations, both Mary and Sylvia co-opt some of the authority of medical professionalism for themselves. Sinclair contrasts Sylvia with her "luxury, beauty, power and prestige," with Mary, who is characterized by her "modern attitude and her common-sense,"[96] which in an unpublished draft Sinclair described more specifically as her

"her science and her common-sense."[97] Mary's health-related knowledge becomes legitimated as Sinclair imbues it with the authority of scientific truth. This medical wisdom confers a unique kind of power to Mary that, in turn, contributes to Sylvia's empowerment when she encourages Sylvia to become further educated about her health.

Because of his recognition of a patriarchal culture of medicine, Sinclair emphasizes how women oppressed by it should not be morally condemned. Consider the character of Claire Lepage, who contracted a venereal disease from Douglas before Sylvia married him—and who appears pleased that he is now infecting Sylvia. At first glance, Sinclair seems to cast Claire as morally corrupt and treacherous, a counterpoint to Mary who responsibly tries to protect Sylvia's health. Claire informs Mary that she knew Douglas had exposed Sylvia to venereal disease, and she asks, "Why should I have it, and she get off?"[98] Yet, Claire argues that her perspective should not be morally judged, adding, "You think I'm as bad as any woman on the street. Very well then, I speak for my class."[99] Sinclair implies that Claire's resentment results from being stifled by a patriarchal system. Claire suggests that she had always intended to punish Douglas and his future children, but although this stance seems ruthless, Sinclair refuses to portray Claire as simply evil. She recalls that she once tried to "trap" Douglas—resonating with Sinclair's idea of marriage as a potential "trap" noted in *Physical Culture*—and in so doing "to get his child in spite of him."[100] However, Claire later laments, "I found that the surgeons had cut me up, and I could never have a child."[101] Claire experienced something akin to forced sterilization. Although the reference is brief, it reveals that patriarchal medical violence—the very kind of abuse the novel critiques—is the fundamental source of Claire's rage. The United States has a long history of eugenic sterilization, beginning with a 1907 Indiana law, followed by similar measures in thirty states and continuing well into the twentieth century. Claire's account exposes these forms of medical violence which Sylvia initially seeks to conceal. Because Claire has been forced to confront the ramifications of patriarchal medicine in ways that Douglas never has, Sinclair invites readers to empathize with her rebellion against oppressive expectations that confine her and jeopardize her health. Moreover, Claire's defiance foreshadows Sylvia's own rebellion: for instance, when Sylvia's aunt advises her to conceal her anger and dress nicely, Sylvia retorts, "A pretty frock, and a seething volcano underneath! That is your idea of a woman's life!" Both Claire and Sylvia challenge conventional expectations regarding domesticity and maternity when their autonomy is compromised.

This kind of emotional repulsion that leads to Claire's rebellion and that gradually leads Sylvia to reject her husband is bestowed with a kind of scientific legitimacy. Sinclair privileges evidence-based, medical rationalism as the foundation for women's health, blending an account of scientific authority with representations of anti-patriarchal rage. In fact, he presents men's sexual behavior rather than women's as irrational. Mary comes to believe that she is perceived as "the mad women who were just then rising to horrify the respectability of England,"[102] and later Douglas refers to Mary as Sylvia's "mad woman friend."[103] When Perrin expresses concern that Sylvia might separate from her husband upon learning the truth about her disease, Mary counters this proposition by noting that Sylvia herself not the "hysterical type."[104] When Gibson contends Mary is "talking madness" and that Sylvia would become "hysterical" if informed of the truth, Mary asserts, she has the "coolest head of anyone I know" and notes, "I do not think of any man I would trust to take a fully rational attitude in the end."[105] Rather than accepting myths of women's hysteria, Mary implies that men's reckless sexual behavior is akin to a kind of madness, and instead champions the protection of women's physical health through scientific reason.

Refuting the notion that knowledge of venereal disease renders patients hysterical, Sinclair insists that knowledge of medical facts will actively promote psychological clarity and empowerment. While Perrin fears that Sylvia's independence would lead her to hysteria, Sinclair depicts Sylvia's rational management of her sexual health as a form of empowerment. When she declares that she will refuse her husband until their health is restored, Sylvia explains that she will withhold intimacy from him, and observes, "it seemed utterly impossible to make him realize what I felt . . . It wasn't only a physical thing, I think; it was an affront on his pride, a denial of this authority."[106] She notes, further, that she will resist his advances "until I have got this disease out of my mind, as well as out of my body; until I know that there is no possibility of either of us having it, to give to the other."[107] Sylvia's realizations are about the effects of venereal disease on the body but also on the mind, and in response, Sinclair portrays the kind of scientific rationalism that the doctors in the novel see as an exclusively masculinist quality being rerouted, through Sylvia's own approach, toward protecting women's physical health and psychological well-being.

Sinclair was acutely aware that medical information about venereal disease was often kept secret, creating an aura of mystery around the disease that was itself dangerous. Early in the novel, Sylvia exclaims—linking the medical profession with a cult of secrecy—"All these doctors—this mystery—this vagueness!"[108] She later acknowledges that she had read "something in a magazine" and remarks, "I thought that—that possibly my fiancé—that someone ought to ask him, you understand."[109] But in addition to this general reference to popular culture signified by the magazine, and the response from Sylvia as she describes something she is only vaguely aware of, in sentence fragments, Sinclair underscores the importance of official medical sources in accruing information. Sylvia eventually visits a medical bookstore, where she pretends to be a physician to access books about sexual health, and then puts this official medical knowledge to insurgent ends. Though Douglas threatens to burn her books, she strategically uses the information she has gleaned from them to justify rejecting him, as she realizes he has jeopardized both her own and her child's health.

Just as Sylvia co-opts some medical authority for herself, Sinclair also provides his readers with medical wisdom as the author of *Sylvia's Marriage*. In unpublished draft material for *Sylvia's Marriage*, Sinclair's intention for the novel to be a kind of "medical book" becomes evident. Sinclair himself not only endorses Mary's and Sylvia's growing medical wisdom but sought to pass it on to his readers. In this unpublished draft, Sinclair wrote about this process of transmitting medical information through the form of the novel:

> "You who read what I have written here—you will blush, perhaps—if you are reading aloud you will hesitate. And yet, I ask you, are not these things true? Are they not things that every man knows to be true? And have I not written of them honestly? You will say they belong somewhere else but in a story. But where? I ask. In medical books? That is to say, they belong in books where they will never be read by the people who need them! No, I say—the books in which they belong are the books which are read."[110]

By drawing a parallel between medical textbooks and fiction, and noting that fiction would reach a wider audience, Sinclair defended his use of a popular and accessible form to promote women's sexual health. For Sinclair,

Sylvia's Marriage was both a work of fiction and a form of progressive sexual health education.

Within the novel, an educated, informed approach to sexual health becomes the basis for Sylvia's decision to reject her husband and patriarchy more generally. Throughout the novel, Sinclair prefigures Sylvia's realization about the perils of venereal disease by insisting that women afflicted with venereal disease are not immoral and instead, he places the blame for its spread on men. At one point, although Sylvia considers venereal disease a "bad disease," Mary explains that while it is indeed "a very bad disease," if one were to assume that only "bad people" contract it, "one should recognize that most men take the chance of getting it; yet they are cruel enough to despise those upon whom misfortune falls."[111] Throughout *Sylvia's Marriage*, Sinclair enumerates the staggering number of venereal disease cases affecting patients across the nation and in so doing emphasizes it is a social issue rather than the result of individual failings. Mary recounts hearing a college professor state that "in his opinion eighty-five per cent of the men students at his university were infected with some venereal disease,"[112] and exclaims, "stop and think . . . ten thousand blind children every year! A hundred thousand women under the surgeon's knife! Millions of women going to pieces with slowly creeping diseases of which they never hear the names!"[113] Later, Mary cites these figures to persuade Douglas to confess that he transmitted gonorrhea to Sylvia, suggesting that she will not be angry once she realizes that his actions are produced by a patriarchal system—that is, "when she has . . . been made to realize that you are no more guilty than other men in your class—that you have done no worse than all of them . . ."[114] Sylvia's realization about the need to leave her husband echoes these earlier moments. She calls attention to the many women who experience threats to their sexual health and independence, coming to understand she "suffered with all the millions of women who gave themselves night after night without love."[115] Sylvia's decision to leave Douglas becomes positioned as an act of rebellion against a much broader assault on women's health.

In portraying this separation, Sinclair rejected the moralistic approach to marriage that some physicians promoted in their views about divorce and aligned himself with more progressive medical views about the matter. Exemplifying a more conservative view, Philadelphia physician Robert Willson noted in 1906 that although reliable data on how often venereal disease led to divorce was lacking, the medical profession had long been aware of the phenomenon: "I read from the national census," he noted, "that during twenty years... we have recorded 328,716 broken homes. How many of these were ruptured because of the husband's infection of the wife, no one will ever know! Perhaps it is as well that no one ever should. Every physician knows of more than one such instance, and one is enough to set manhood aflame."[116] Willson presented divorce as unspeakable and shameful, much like venereal disease itself, viewing divorce as a tragic symptom of venereal disease in marriages. Alternatively, Prince A. Morrow advocated more sympathetically for acceptance of divorce in cases involving venereal disease as a mechanism of self-protection and empowerment: "no other commentary," he noted, "upon the intolerable situations created by the introduction of these diseases into the family is needed than the fact that so many women, loyal to the highest ideals of marriage, devoted to home and family, are driven to the divorce courts as a refuge. No one can condemn a self-respecting woman for separating from a man who has dishonored her with a shameful disease."[117] In *Sylvia's Marriage*, Sinclair resists constraining attitudes about compulsory domesticity and instead valorizes Sylvia's rejection of her husband as an act of rebellion that promotes sexual autonomy. When Douglas attempts to persuade Sylvia of the "duties of marriage—the preserving of the home, wives submitting themselves to their husbands, and so on," a view that resonates with Sylvia's doctors' perception of maternal duties, Sylvia simply retorts, "it is not only the tragedy of my blind child—it's that you have driven me to hate you."[118] Sinclair, as noted, had mentioned in *Physical Culture*, that the "first duty" of a potential husband was to protect his future wife's health, but Douglas refuses to take this kind of duty to heart, which leads Sylvia to resist him. In portraying Sylvia rejecting and separating from her husband, Sinclair resists the dictates of compulsory domesticity, instead privileging the right to sexual health, even when it leads to marital discord and potential separation.

Some readers were critical of *Sylvia's Marriage*'s didactic agenda and considered whether or not it had been effective as a novel. One reviewer argued that the novel contained too much medical detail, trying to serve an educational purpose at the expense of emotional engagement. This reviewer remarked that "psychology should be more important to the novelist than a medical dictionary" and further questioned Sinclair's statistics: "I question the inference which Sinclair draws that nine men out of ten are affected with venereal disease... I have no way of verifying his statistics, and I doubt whether he has. But they do not appeal to me as being plausible, and right or wrong, I believe they will cause skepticism in many minds and tend to discredit the rest of his work."[119] Nonetheless, setting aside questions of statistical accuracy, Sinclair's commitment to an evidence-oriented aesthetic enabled him to strategically control, manipulate, and subvert conventional love plots that minimized the risks of venereal disease. In this respect, despite some of the reservations expressed, this reviewer found the novel effective, anticipating that it would help prevent the spread of venereal disease, especially stopping men from infecting innocent women. He noted that *Sylvia's Marriage* taught readers that "men who lead dissolute lives expose themselves to terrible and almost inescapable physical consequences; that many men who thus become infected with venereal diseases have enough of the demon in them to persist in marriage with innocent and unsuspecting women ... and that the horrible danger to which girls and women are exposed by being willfully kept in ignorance of these pitfalls of sex life ought—in the name of all that is clean, just, and honorable—to be stopped."[120]

In an article for *The Nation*, *Sylvia's Marriage* was characterized as a "pamphlet, and a very severe and courageous one too"; the "construction of 'Sylvia's Marriage,'" the author noted, "its atmosphere and characters are all subordinated to one definite end—the exposure of the 'conspiracy of silence concerning sexual disease.'" But the reviewer complained that "the psychological structure of the book is superfluous. Sylvia is not a person but the voice of a cause. The great novelist can combine the two; the inspired zealot and reformer, on the other hand, can present his case for more efficiently without introducing at all the distracting elements of the novel form."[121] However, the psychological aspects of *Sylvia's Marriage*, like those in Gilman's *The Crux*, including the extensive discussions of characters' repulsion from particular men, are in fact critical to their aims in demonstrating that sexual health is a critical component of women's marital rights.

After writing *Sylvia's Marriage*, Sinclair would continue to discuss venereal disease and its relationship with women's rights in his later writing. In a 1918 issue of *A Monthly Magazine*, Sinclair indicated he still thought of syphilis and gonorrhea as diseases about which "we know so much, and do almost nothing!"[122] For his part, Sinclair continued to educate himself about these diseases by researching the latest medical developments. With this information, he looked for ways to curb their spread by advocating for careful marital decisions and the dissemination of accurate medical information with a particular emphasis on protecting women's health.

However, as becomes apparent from an unpublished manuscript written around or shortly after 1918, for Sinclair this task could be linked to a eugenic mission. Speaking of a "percentage of venereal diseases" that he understood to be "appalling," he criticized legal protections for prostitution in the following terms: "Can we deliberately take the backward step of legislating for increased promiscuous intercourse, that vast distributor of venereal diseases?" he asked. "What race improvement will follow from such a legislation?" Though he noted it could hamper the "happiness of the individual" and the "legacy" to the individual "child," he failed to disentangle these risks from the kinds of perceived risks of national "degeneration" that Gilman also feared.[123]

In his self-help book *The Book of Life* (1921), Sinclair examined the threat posed by venereal disease, asking, "What are the consequences of these diseases? The consequences are frightful suffering, not merely to persons guilty of immorality, but to innocent persons." Citing Prince A. Morrow's research, he noted that "ten per cent of all wives are infected with venereal disease by their husbands; he estimates that thirty per cent of all the infected women in New York were wives who had got the disease from their husbands."[124] Writing again in defense of a monogamous ideal, Sinclair argued that sexual contact outside of marriage must be limited: "I know, of course, that there are prophylactics, and the army and navy present statistics to show that they succeed in a great proportion of cases. But if you are one of those persons in whose case they don't succeed, you will find the statistics a cold source of comfort to you."[125] Instead of relying solely on physical prophylaxis, Sinclair advocated for social prophylaxis through the minimization of sexual encounters. While privileging monogamy as an ideal might seem conservative and moralistic, for Sinclair it was linked to the valuation of women's health. In fact Sinclair viewed the ideal of monogamy as serving a similar function as allowing for divorce in some instances: both monogamy as an ideal and divorce as an option could be connected to women's self-empowerment and health.

Sinclair's account in *The Book of Life* of a young couple navigating sexual health concerns encapsulates how, in his view, scientific reason could inform marriage plans: "John and Mary go to the altar, or to the justice of the peace, and John says: 'With all my worldly goods I thee endow.' But the formula is incomplete; it ought to read: 'And likewise with the fruits of my wild oats.' Marriage is a contract wherein each of the contracting parties agrees to share whatever pathogenic bacteria the other may have or acquire; surely, therefore, the contract involves a right of each party to have a say as to how many chances of infection the other shall incur." By presenting marriage in these new medical terms, Sinclair defamiliarized the institution. In particular, he aligned the protection of women's health with rational, scientific thinking about disease—contrasting this with men's convoluted romantic emotions and risky sexual lives. Continuing his anecdote about John and Mary, Sinclair observed: "John goes off on a business trip, and is lonesome, and meets an agreeable widow, and figures to himself that there is very little chance that so charming a person can be dangerous. But maybe Mary wouldn't agree with his calculations; maybe Mary would not consider it a part of the marriage bargain that she should take the diseases of the agreeable widow ... How can any thinking person deny that John has thus committed an act of treason to Mary?"[126] Here, just as was the case with Sinclair's emphasis on scientific rationalism and women's rights in *Sylvia's Marriage*, Sinclair positioned John's "lonesomeness"—constituted by his sad, undisciplined feelings—as a threat to a rational, "thinking" approach to romance that prioritizes women's health.

For H. L. Mencken, this rational and scientific approach to romance appeared humorous. In his play *Asepsis* (1913), he satirized what he viewed as the excessive preoccupation with venereal disease among young couples. In one scene, a clergyman informs an engaged couple that they will enter "holy matrimony" only after "due surgical precautions ... reverently, cleanly, sterilely, soberly, scientifically, and with the nearest practicable approach to bacteriological purity ... Into this laudable and non-infectious state these two persons present come now to be joined and quarantined. If any man can show just cause, either clinically or microscopically, why they may be safely sutured together, let him now forward with his charts, slides and cultures, or else hereafter hold his peace."[127] Mencken interwove medical and romantic language in order to ridicule reformers' scientific explanations of desire, which he saw as absurd.

For Gilman and Sinclair, though, applying a scientific perspective to marriage and love was essential, not in order to promote general moralistic notions of purity but rather to promote women's health. They not only portrayed characters being educated about the risks of venereal disease to women's health, but they also sought to educate their readers about these risks. Gilman, whose own work was overtly didactic, wrote in a review of

Sylvia's Marriage that it effectively exposed "the terrible results of gonorrhea, as well as the danger of ignorance, and the conspiracy of silence by which offenders are protected," though she noted that "judged by the best of Mr. Sinclair's work, it is not a good novel, but a sincere and vigorous effort to expose a very real evil . . ."[128] Yet Sinclair, like Gilman herself, combined elements of medical didacticism with love plots riddled with emotional tension. While the physician characters in *Sylvia's Marriage* claim scientific rigor as a masculinist characteristic, Mary and Sylvia challenge these assumptions by promoting women's health from deeply scientific perspectives. As Gilman draws from medical science while attending to matters of feeling, Sinclair depicts Mary and Sylvia as embracing their own factual, medical approach even to deeply emotional aspects of conflicts over sexual health. Both writers strove to interweave medical expertise with powerful, rebellious sentiments, as they protested against patriarchal attitudes shaping public health that were both unscientific and unfeeling. However, their investments in state regulation to protect white, middle-class marriages compromised their missions, making it all the more critical to envision possibilities for radically inclusive and truly liberational narratives of autonomy, choice, and sexual health.

CHAPTER FOUR

Disability, Euthanasia, Survival

THE AUTHOR JACK LONDON held that dying could be both a right and a duty. In a 1913 issue of the *Medical Review of Reviews*, London was quoted as supporting euthanasia on the grounds of individual rights: "Man... possesses but one freedom, namely the anticipating of the day of his death... Should collective man (the state) rob individual man of this one freedom?" He then answered his own question unequivocally, writing: "I believe in euthanasia. I believe that the state should make legal the painless ending of helpless incurables who desire to die."[1] While London ostensibly championed an individual's right to die in a manner of their own choosing, he was particularly concerned with a group he labeled "helpless incurables," a phrase that underscores how stigmatizing views of disability underpinned his argument. At a time when debates about euthanasia were increasingly prominent, London's fiction further reveals how stigmatizing views of disability informed these discussions. In his earlier short story "The Law of Life" (1901), London appears to accept the notion of a duty to die. The story follows a blind member of a nomadic tribe who is abandoned by his community and gradually accepts his fate as being part of a natural order: "it was easy. All men must die. He did not complain. It was the way of life, and it was just... it was the law of all flesh. Nature was not kindly to the flesh. She had no concern for that concrete thing called the individual. Her interest lay in the species, the race."[2] Here, London stages a naturalist logic of euthanasia, which the protagonist internalizes. A key feature of naturalism, a genre deeply influenced by medical and pseudo-scientific theories, has been its emphasis on individuals' fates being shaped or predetermined by heredity and environment, often culminating in degeneration and decline. In this story, disability is presented as rendering a character "naturally" fit only for death, reinforcing the stigmatizing assumptions embedded in London's argument. In presenting a premature death as something done for the sake of the "species," London portrayed death not only as an individual liberty—as per his statement about death as a kind of "freedom"- but, troublingly, as a social responsibility.

Rosemarie Garland-Thomson refers to the desire to eliminate disability from the social body that was prevalent in early twentieth-century progressivist politics as the "cultural logic of euthanasia." She illustrates this concept through Herman Melville's novella "Bartleby, the Scrivener" (1856), a work composed before euthanasia became widely debated within the medical community. Though the story makes no explicit mention of euthanasia it does address disability, illness, care, and death. In "Bartleby," an unnamed lawyer employs a copyist whom he labels "deranged" and "incurable"—an implicitly medicalized characterization—and who chooses to die. As Garland-Thomson notes, Bartleby's society views him as "flawed, in need of regularization, and ultimately—if not curable—expendable" revealing the early contours of a kind of prejudice toward disability that would later undergird pro-euthanasia arguments.[3]

By the turn of the twentieth century, as debates over "mercy killing" became increasingly visible, the stigmatization of disability that Melville critiqued in "Bartleby" surfaced in both medicine and popular culture. While the idea of a "good death" dates back much earlier, it was in this period that euthanasia emerged as a distinctly medical phenomenon. During the antebellum period, the term still connoted a peaceful death granted by God, but by later in the nineteenth century, it came to refer more narrowly to the physician's deliberate hastening of death. This development paralleled medicine's expanding authority over death itself, following the isolation of morphine from opium and the discovery of anesthetics.[4] By the beginning of the new century, Americans were discussing euthanasia more openly than ever, with the topic generating substantial debate among medical professionals and the general public, as well as heightened coverage in the mass media and in literature.

Much of the discussion about physician-assisted death centered on those deemed physically or mentally disabled. These stances were rooted in troubling assumptions about the supposed burden of disability, both to disabled individuals and to society as a whole. Though proponents of euthanasia claimed to be motivated by compassion for disabled patients, early arguments for a right to die rooted in benevolence often thinly veiled discriminatory assumptions. Framing euthanasia as a merciful solution was frequently paired with an ulterior motive: to alleviate the presumed burden their existence placed on communities and even the nation as a whole. Arguments for euthanasia often conflated the sense of a right to die with a perceived social responsibility to eliminate those deemed unfit for life from taxing the nation, as was noted by commentators and doctors who criticized pro-euthanasia arguments as a threat to both medical ethics and the profession's public reputation. In 1903, for instance, a contributor to the *Journal of the American Medical Association* denounced the misguided "philanthropist" who advocates speeding the death of "invalids," insisting that doctors had "no right to trifle with a human life or shorten it by a second."[5] As physician Abraham Jacobi further cautioned, in 1912, normalizing euthanasia would undermine medicine's status as a "respectable calling."[6] One widely publicized example of the kind of violent cultural logic these commentors critiqued is to be found in the case of Harry Haiselden, a surgeon at Chicago's German American Hospital. Haiselden not only refused to treat disabled infants but, in at least one instance, deliberately ended a newborn's life.[7] In 1915, he advised Anna Bollinger that her disabled baby would be better off if he did not perform a lifesaving surgery on him. The resulting death of the Bollinger's baby became a national sensation, and Haiselden soon appeared in a propaganda film titled *Are You Fit to Marry?* (1916), co-written with Jack Lait. The film dramatizes the convoluted logic underlying Haiselden's practice: it follows a wealthy man named Claude, who inherits "the blood taint of an indiscreet ancestor"—a "servant . . . an unclean creature."[8] Though a doctor warns him otherwise, Claude marries Anna, and their disabled child is born. Anna then sees a vision from God of the boy's grim future if allowed to live: He is ostracized, becomes violent, and murders the doctor who refused to end his life. Rather than casting euthanasia itself as lethal, *Are You Fit to Marry?* egregiously frames disability as the true danger. Anna decides to encourage the doctor to euthanize him. The ideas within *Are You Fit to Marry?* were not an anomaly but, unfortunately, held a broad base of support, including that of prominent figures such as Lillian Wald and Helen Keller, as well as the many parents who wrote to Haiselden requesting that he euthanize their disabled children.[9]

While proponents of euthanasia positioned the disabled as menacing to the social body and their premature deaths as natural, authors such as Edith Wharton, Stephen Crane, and Dalton Trumbo, responded by presenting euthanasia itself as dangerous and unnatural. In particular, they argued against any notion of a duty to die. Although they did not always provide explicit denunciations of physician-assisted death in general, and in some instances even recognized individuals' right to die, they called attention to the stigmatization of disability that shaped arguments for euthanasia. The authors I discuss in this chapter treated medical attitudes toward disability with ambivalence: while recognizing that certain disabilities do require medical care, they sought changes to conventional medical understandings of disability. Well before the organized disability-rights movement emerged in the late twentieth century, these authors recognized the urgent need for medical professionals to safeguard disabled patients' interests. Their fiction challenged a prevailing view of disabled lives as lives not worth living and specifically pointed to social forces that were debilitating patients,[10] slowly killing them, or relegating them to the status of being perceived as already dead. They unmasked the deceptive euphemisms of euthanasia arguments. They exposed the underlying illogic of the notion that a premature death would be natural, instead realistically portraying the suffering caused by debilitating injuries and disabled patients' own desires, which could entail death wishes but also, however paradoxically, an insistence on survival. In so doing, they worked to untether perceptions of disability from images of death and doom.

Survival

In *The Monster* (1898), Stephen Crane situated euthanasia within a broader network of questions about life, death, and disability, depicting a proposed act of "mercy killing" as a misguided attempt to shield a community from a disabled individual perceived as a monstrous threat. The novella portrays Henry Johnson, a coachman working for Dr. Ned Trescott in the town of Whilomville, who saves Trescott's son Jimmie from a fire that erupts in Trescott's home. In the process, Henry's face becomes disfigured. A judge, Hagenthorpe, subsequently recommends that Henry be euthanized on the grounds that his disability renders him fit only to die. Ned, however, rejects Hagenthorpe's decision, and Henry survives.[11] Throughout the novella, references to euthanasia are interwoven with explorations of life, death, and disability more generally.

At the beginning of *The Monster*, Stephen Crane offers a telling detail that foreshadows later events. Jimmie, Ned's son, has damaged a peony and attempts to "stand it on its pins, resuscitated, but the spine of it was hurt, and it would only hang limply from his hand. Jim could do no reparation."[12] This minor scene of injury and incomplete recovery prefigures the novella's larger questions concerning life, harm, and death.[13] Indeed, *The Monster* as a whole centers on two acts of lifesaving care—Henry Johnson's rescue of Jimmie and Ned's lifesaving protection of Henry—that can only partially address the long history of collectively inflicted injury on disabled patients and populations.

The account of Henry's survival following the fire in Ned's home poses a challenge to ableist assumptions, one that anticipates Crane's critique of euthanasia. Henry is badly hurt when he rushes into Ned's laboratory to save Jimmie. At first, he appears resigned to death, which Crane likens to "a most perfect slavery," hinting that Henry internalizes the belief his life is disposable. In fact, he is portrayed as "bending his mind" to this slavery, as Crane presents a critique of debilitation's effects on psychology.[14] Though at first Henry "had almost given up all idea of escaping from the burning house, and with it the desire," he finally resists this self-sacrificial mindset and recalls a hidden stairway, prompting "the old frantic terror" that spurs him back toward survival, as he becomes "no longer creature to the flames."[15] This vaguely defined "old" fear predates the sudden emergence of the fire, suggesting that what haunts Henry is not just the imminent danger he faces, but his social marginalization more fundamentally.

Later, from Ned's perspective, Hagenthorpe will seem to associate euthanasia with an "old problem," as the kind of language used to describe Henry's resolute choice to live, through the reference to the "old frantic terror" that spurs him toward self-protection, becomes distorted into a rationale for ending his life.[16] After the fire, when Hagenthorpe first raises the possibility of euthanasia to Ned, he does so in an ambivalent, suggestive manner that masks euthanasia's violence. He at first simply asks, "Who knows" in a "deep tone" that gave his words "an elusive kind of significance."[17] Hagenthorpe prefaces his recommendation by recounting a version of the *Frankenstein* story, informing Ned that Henry "will be your creation, you understand. He is purely your creation.... He is dead. You are restoring him to life. You are making him, and he will be a monster, and with no mind."[18] In claiming the intended recipient of euthanasia is already dead, Hagenthorpe's comment closely parallels euthanasia arguments at the time, including, for instance, perceptions of John Bollinger, whom Harry Haiselden argued had a "tiny brain" and therefore "was not a live thing—but a dead and fearsome ounce or two of jelly," maintaining that "those who have no brains—their blank and awful existence cannot be called Life."[19] By thinking about disabled patients' as being somehow already dead, supporters of euthanasia minimized their capacity to suffer, suggesting the act had negligible moral stakes. In *The Monster*, Crane similarly shows Hagenthorpe describing Henry as already dead, as he diminishes the brutality of the proposal of euthanasia while conversely portraying the decision to actively "make" Henry—which would really mean letting him live—as a cruel act.

Hagenthorpe's view further obscures what would amount to murder. Associating euthanasia with a mysterious, vague problem, he sidesteps the specific realities of disabled embodiment in favor of sweeping, abstract moralism. He blames Ned for "performing a questionable charity" by saving Henry, labeling this one of the "blunders of virtue." Yet such notions of charity and ethics deflect attention from the underlying fact that he is advocating for killing a disabled patient. At the turn of the twentieth century, proponents of euthanasia often described the act as letting individuals die rather than actively ending their lives. In *The Monster*, Hagenthorpe uses a similarly vague approach, telling Ned that "no one wants to advance such ideas, but somehow I think that that poor fellow ought to die."[20] He articulates a superficial reluctance, noting "it is hard for a man to know what to do"[21]—as though he has not already made up his mind. Such indirection, vagueness, and feigned uncertainty shroud the violence of his proposal.

In *The Monster*, Crane portrays Henry's suffering as a result of unnatural cruelty while implying that euthanasia would extend this violence. As Jacqueline Goldsby explains, Crane wrote *The Monster*, in part, in response to a lynching that took place in Port Jervis, New York, in 1892, when a mob murdered Robert Lewis, an African American coachman accused of raping a white woman. This history of brutal violence reverberates through Crane's portrayal of Henry's injury. Crane insists that it is not "Nature" but rather the surrounding community that has given up on and directly debilitated Henry. Even the fire in which Henry is injured is described as having "been well planned, as if by professional revolutionists,"[22] suggesting an intentional scheme rather than an impersonal force. Further, the smoke is said to be "alive with envy, hatred, and malice."[23] By personifying the fire as a sentient, hostile presence, Crane links the flames to the community's vicious hatred. Like Hagenthorpe's discussion of euthanasia, the fire is strongly associated with a history of targeted animosity and calculated, premeditated violence.

In this context, a particularly pernicious element of Hagenthorpe's argument is how he defines what is natural. He insists Henry is effectively dead because "nature has very evidently given him up."[24] This stance not only positions Ned's lifesaving actions as a violation of the natural order, but it also obscures the social causes of Henry's vulnerability. His debility arises not from an inescapable biological fate but rather from deliberate, damaging human interventions. Unlike the notion in Jack London's "The Law of Life" of "nature" punishing an individual, leading to disability and death, Crane critiques Hagenthorpe's naturalistic language through his distinctly realist aesthetic. Generally, Crane's work does exhibit naturalist characteristics, and *Maggie: A Girl of the Streets* (1893), with its narrative of poverty and prostitution culminating in death, offers a classic example. However, Crane also often subverts and ironically complicates such naturalistic plots.[25] In particular, *The Monster* complicates the determinism often associated with naturalism as Crane realistically emphasizes the causes and consequences of human behavior and choice rather than a predestined course of "nature." This distinction becomes especially important in the context of a doctor-patient story given how profoundly medicine shapes cultural ideas about what is natural.[26]

In addition, further reinforcing the danger of devaluing disabled lives, a diffuse kind of lethal force continues to hang over the story after Henry's injury. Although Henry ultimately avoids euthanasia, the necropolitical[27] mindset underlying it persists. Ned's efforts are insufficient: even though Henry, Jimmie, and Ned survive the fire, the town still considers them on the brink of death. The firemen who carry their cots are likened to "foot-men to death," while the onlookers make a "subtle obeisance to this august dignity derived from three prospective graves."[28] A bystander, confronted, exclaims that while these individuals might not already be dead, "they'll die sure." Rumors come to circulate that Henry, Jimmie, and Ned have all perished. When it becomes evident that they have survived, Henry—unlike Ned and Jimmie—remains locked in the community's imagination as already dead or fated to an early death. Though Crane notes that Ned's burns are "not vitally important" and Jimmie's "life was undoubtedly safe," Henry, according to the community's perception of him, "could not live."[29] Other patients at Hagenthorpe's residence warn that he is "doomed," and a false obituary in the next day's newspaper draws belated pity from townspeople who wish they had aided him "when he was alive."[30] Despite Henry's having escaped both the fire and Hagenthorpe's proposal of euthanasia, the townspeople continue to regard him as marked by death. Local children see him as an embodiment of mourning: his singing strikes them as "mournful and slow," a tune with "the power of a funeral."[31] Alek Williams and his wife, who care for Henry after he is injured, treat him as one would a bereaved individual "in church at funerals," bracing themselves for some "calamity" that is "pealing and deadly."[32] An especially telling moment occurs when the children sing a taunting refrain of "never die"[33] between the false report of Henry's death and the revelation that he is still alive; this refrain becomes cruelly ironic in a community that already perceives Henry as inevitably doomed. What is more, Henry's community associates him not only with being doomed but with being a violent threat to others: as one character remarks, "everybody that's seen him say they were frightened almost to death."[34] As is the case with the propaganda film *Are You Fit to Marry?*, in which disability would be caricatured as menacing and even lethal, in "The Monster," the Whilomville community views Henry as both already dead and dangerous to the living, rather than understanding the threat of euthanasia is the real danger in question.

A seemingly peripheral scene illustrates this dynamic when, upon learning of Henry's injury, a barber named Reifsnyder overhears a railway engineer commenting on Ned's choice to let Henry live. "Oh, he should have let him die," the engineer declares. Reifsnyder counters, "How can you let a man die?" only to be told, "By letting him die, you chump." At first, Reifsnyder appears to pose a general ethical question—how could one possibly allow another human being to die? Yet when he rephrases it as "How can you let a man die when he has done so much for you?" he implicitly refers to how Henry saved Jimmie from the fire. In this sense, he reveals how the community's well-being and even their very lives are in fact dependent on Henry's own act of care, even as Henry is cruelly equated with death in the community's imagination.

At the same time, Ned's efforts at saving Henry present a defiant challenge to the argument for euthanasia. After the fire, builders quickly erect a new house on Ned's property, the "black mass" of the old one barely cooled before construction begins.[35] It "sprung upward at a fabulous rate," Crane writes, "like a magical composition born of the ashes . . . ," and he is quick to move in "his new books and instruments and medicines there."[36] This image of Ned's medical profession rising out of the fire aligns Ned's lifesaving mission with a hopeful, forward-looking vision of medicine through these motifs of vitality amidst ruinous violence. In an analogous way, Henry's continued presence—made possible by both his own self-protection and Ned's medical care—challenges the community's insistence that his disability dooms him. Between the false reports of Henry's death and the ongoing references to him in terms of death-related imagery, Crane simply writes: "Later in the day Miss Bella Farragut, of No. 7 Watermelon Alley, announced that she had been engaged to marry Mr. Henry Johnson." The shift from rumors of Henry's death to news of his engagement is abrupt, and there is not much in the way of an explanation for Henry's survival after this moment. While pro-euthanasia arguments in the novella are vague, abstract, and senseless, Henry's refusal to succumb to a premature death speaks for itself—directly and concretely. In relaying this, Crane suggests that neither the worth of disabled life nor the fact of survival requires further justification, and in so doing, he points clearly and realistically toward a future beyond convoluted arguments for euthanasia.

Life, Death, and Disability

Following the publication of "The Monster," euthanasia reemerged in American fiction within Edith Wharton's *The Fruit of the Tree* (1907). Wharton had been drawn to the notion of a peaceful death but remained concerned that this ethical stance could be abused. She believed that end-of-life matters—such as suicide and physician-assisted death—should be less taboo. In a 1901 letter to her friend Sara ("Sally") Norton regarding her mother's passing, Wharton described it as a merciful release from suffering: "She had been hopelessly ill for fourteen months, paralyzed and unconscious nearly a year," yet "it was one of those cases in which it seems that life—that kind of life—might go on for years."[37] A few years later, in December 1904, Wharton sought the advice of Dr. Francis Kinnicutt on how Lily Bart—her protagonist in *The House of Mirth*—might end her life. Referring obliquely to Lily, Wharton wrote, "A friend of mine . . . has made up her mind to commit suicide . . . & has asked me to find out . . . the most painless & least unpleasant method of effacing herself."[38] She then clarified her intentions for the novel: "I have heroine to get rid of, and want some points on the best way of disposing her." Wondering which "soporific" or "nerve-calming drug" a young, anxious socialite would take to end her life,

Wharton asked about both the drug's likely effects and "how she would feel and look toward the end." In addition, in a 1910 letter to John Hugh Smith, Wharton underscored her conviction about the importance of a "peaceful death," calling it "infinitely better than a gradual failure of body or mind."[39]

Wharton's emphasis on a peaceful death led her to argue that, in certain cases, the right to die should be both recognized and facilitated by the medical professions. In a 1905 letter to Sara Norton, Wharton wrote of Ethel Cram, a friend who lost consciousness after a pony-cart accident in July of that year. When a motorcar startled her horse, Cram was thrown from the cart and fractured her skull, remaining unconscious until she died two months later. Reflecting on how physicians artificially prolonged Cram's life, Wharton referenced an 1899 article titled "The Natural Right to a Natural Death," by jurist Simeon Baldwin, then president of the American Bar Association. Baldwin advocated legalizing euthanasia and recounted a cancer patient's plea ("They will not let me die; I want to die"), insisting that a suffering life "prolonged in hopeless misery by medical art, against the sufferer's will . . . when Nature, or let us rather say, that God whose voice is Nature has plainly called him away" was both cruel and unnatural.[40] Wharton responded, "I have thought often of that article of Dr. Baldwin's during these terrible weeks!—I am sure I should have the 'triste courage,' in such a case, to let life ebb out quietly—should not you?"[41]

Later, in a 1908 letter to Sara Norton, Wharton wrote about a neighbor named Hartmann Kuhn, who suffered from a painful illness. Wharton remarked that "if I had morphia in reach, as she has, how quickly I'd cut the knot!" Commenting on the death of Sara Norton's father, Charles Norton, she confessed: "How I grieve with you, ache for you, poor child, the more perhaps as what you speak of is only partly intelligible, or is not so at all. But if it is a retrospect of wasted, wasteful, pain, oh then how my own joins itself to yours!"[42] This correspondence implies that the Norton family may have aligned their private actions with their public endorsement of euthanasia,[43] and Wharton was offering them her support.

Yet despite Wharton's acceptance of the right to die—a position that arose from her compassion for suffering—in *The Fruit of the Tree* she critiqued the assumptions that often underwrote pro-euthanasia views. Wharton insisted in a letter to the editor Edward Burlingame that her novel was not intended as a "thesis for or against euthanasia."[44] Nevertheless, in it, Wharton clearly unsettled harmful strains of euthanasia rhetoric. Refusing to conflate disability and death, *Fruit of the Tree* focuses on the ethical complexities of medical decisions and emphasizes how certain pro-euthanasia arguments rest on stigmatizing notions of disability. Though Wharton's well-known novels of Old New York society—*The Age of Innocence, The House of Mirth*, and *The Custom of the Country*—may lead readers to regard her as an unlikely commentator on social issues like euthanasia, *The Fruit of the Tree* demonstrates a decidedly sociopolitical engagement. As Karen Weingarten observes, disability in Wharton's work has often been read metaphorically: disability in these readings is understood as a tool for social critique of industrialization and gender roles. Yet she urges readers to also grapple with disability in Wharton's fiction as a tangible reality meriting attention in its own right.[45]

Such a disability-focused reading of *The Fruit of the Tree* can entail examining its seemingly distinct storylines together. In the novel, Wharton creates parallels between the experiences of two patients—Dillon, an industrial worker, and Bessy Westmore, heir to the mills where Dillon is employed—both of whom are deemed to be better off dead when they become disabled. To underscore her critique of prejudiced views about disabled populations, Wharton bridges the disparate subplots of the novel—about euthanasia, reform, and desire—around issues of life, death, and disability. R. W. B. Lewis remarked that *The Fruit of the Tree* contains "too many 'subjects,'" with euthanasia only one among them. While the book's seemingly divergent storylines have perplexed many readers, Wharton interlinks these plots through recurring motifs. Two characters in the novel—Bessy and Dillon—are each deemed worthy or unworthy of life because of their disabilities that render their lives as seemingly useless to others. To illustrate this, Wharton subtly intertwines narratives of medicine and reform. She describes, in one moment, how John Amherst, manager of the industrial factory who is married to Bessy, learns to perceive the mills through "the nurse's eyes."[46] Conversely, she shows how Justine, a nurse at the factory hospital working with John, in confronting Bessy's plight, remembers John's earlier query in the factory hospital—"Don't you ever feel tempted to set a poor devil free?"[47] Industrial reform that fails to address underlying conditions of debilitation, and medical attitudes that fail to acknowledge the value of disabled lives, become associatively entangled, each posing lethal threats even under the guise of care.

CHAPTER FOUR

Although the characters discussing euthanasia appear to act from benevolent motives, closer scrutiny reveals their intentions to be far less innocent. Wharton suggests that within industrial capitalism, both a lack of care and distorted forms of compassionate care itself can be as threatening as overt violence. Early in the novel, John and Justine encounter a worker named Dillon, who has been injured by factory machinery. The mill's overseer attributes Dillon's misfortune to the workers' "carelessness,"[48] yet the other workers insist the real culprit is the mill's unsafe conditions. As John explains to Justine, the carding room is overcrowded in order to "get the maximum of profit out of the minimum of floor-space."[49] By revealing Dillon's injury to be a consequence of exploitive systems rather than individual negligence, Wharton echoes the logic of debilitation seen in "The Monster." But though John views himself as caring and philanthropic, Wharton is skeptical of the shallow sympathy he offers. He treats his workers not as people but as "hands," limiting his empathy to an abstract, dehumanizing vision of industrial labor. As Jennie Kassanoff observes, the term "hands" in *The Fruit of the Tree* reveals the limits of John's idealistic but ultimately impersonal and corporatized thinking about the workers.[50] Early in the novel, when John and Justine stand over Dillon in the factory hospital, John posits to Justine that death for Dillon might be preferable to life: "If I saw the suffering as you see it, and knew the circumstances as I know them. . . ."[51] John reduces him to an object of pity rather than viewing him as a person with intrinsic value. He assumes that Justine, as a nurse, would recognize that euthanasia would be desired, an assumption that is couched in the rhetoric of compassion but that is predicated on the instrumentalization of Dillon's life.

Although Dillon can speak for himself, neither Justine nor John fully acknowledges his agency. One of Dillon's few direct statements is that he wants to return to his family, referring to "four of 'em at home,"[52] yet Justine and John—each convinced they know what is best—overlook this desire. As James Tuttleton notes, an "abstract idealism" pervades their reasoning.[53] Even as both recognize the need for improved working conditions, they fail to see Dillon's individual life as having any value beyond serving a purpose through industrial labor. In this sense, their social-reform rhetoric remains hollow, as they ignore how specific lives—like Dillon's—are affected by the oppressive systems that they only seek to ameliorate to an inadequate extent. Note that Dillon's hand is gravely injured by what Wharton calls a "murderous machine," even as he survives the exploitative labor conditions that are slowly killing him. Wharton shows that these conditions have drained the workers' vitality and leave the industrial slums looking "stone dead," according to Justine.[54] John recognizes that the "deadening toil" of labor saps the workers' vitality, observing their "dull eyes and anaemic skins."[55] Yet, the value of Dillon's already-imperiled life is questioned by both John and Justine as soon as he can no longer work.

In addition, John's insight into the conditions faced by the mill workers is distorted by the way he is enraptured by the very industrial machinery that continues to harm them. In fact, John associates this machinery with life itself. While projecting death onto the workers, John sees the machinery of the mills as akin to a living being: "—he felt a beauty in the ordered activity of the whole intricate organism, in the rhythm of dancing bobbins and revolving cards, the swift continuous outpour of doublers and ribbon-laps, the steady ripple of the long ply-frames, the terrible gnashing play of the looms—all these varying subordinate motions, gathered up into the throb of the great engines which fed the giant's arteries, and were in turn ruled by the invisible action of quick thought and obedient hands, always produced in John a responsive rush of life."[56] The machine is imbued with a kind of vitality—with "arteries," and akin to an "organism" that moves and throbs, depending on the labor of "hands." While living, debilitated people in *Fruit* are treated as malfunctioning machinery, John perceives the machinery of the mills in terms of human embodiment, motion, and life. As such, while Wharton notes that John hated the labor conditions of the mills, his "zeal for his cause was always quickened by the sight of the mills in action."[57] In a way that implies that his dedication to his cause is quite dubious, John sees Dillon as better off dead while encountering the industrial machinery that injured him as enlivening.

A similarly distorted perception of disability surfaces within Justine's perspective when Bessy becomes paralyzed after falling off a horse named Impulse. Justine, who is charged with Bessy's care, administers euthanasia to her and shortly afterward marries John. The exploitation of care is therefore most conspicuous in that Wharton juxtaposes a scene of euthanasia with an ensuing love story, suggesting that Justine is not driven entirely by selfless motives. Though Bessy's life is at first valued more than Dillon's, the perceived value of her life also becomes vulnerable. Unlike Dillon, who is injured by unsafe machinery, Bessy suffers a riding accident brought on by her own recklessness. As opposed to Dillon, who is impoverished,

Bessy is born into wealth. She is viewed by her doctors as inherently worthy of saving. Her life has been lavish—"Life had been poured out to her in generous measure, and she had spilled the precious draught—the few drops remaining in the cup could no longer renew her strength"—and the physicians in charge view the value of her life in similar generous terms.[58] Yet, while Bessy's life is at first valued to a greater extent than that of Dillon, Justine's decision to euthanize Bessy stems from a surge of emotion that compromises her obligations as a nurse. Wharton shows Justine's emotional state gradually intensifying until it erodes her capacity to maintain disinterested professional boundaries. At first, Justine performs her nursing tasks "mechanically," but Bessy's cries eventually strike her not "as the utterance of human pain, but the monotonous whimper of an animal—the kind of sound that a compassionate hand would instinctively crush into silence."[59] Though Justine is sympathetic to Bessy's suffering, her impulse to "crush" this noise is chilling, and combined with the dehumanization associated with animal imagery, it begins to complicate any sense that Justine's act is purely innocent.

Wharton dwells on the compromised nature of Justine's thought process that leads her to this act. From Wharton's correspondence, it is clear that she supported the right to die in some instances. At the same time, in *Fruit* she clearly criticizes the way that pro-euthanasia views can severely distort professionalism. To be sure, the physicians responsible for Bessy's treatment insist on keeping her alive for questionable reasons—as they see an opportunity to advance their professional reputations. Yet Justine also harbors dubious motives for administering a lethal dose of morphine. Wharton depicts her conduct not simply as a merciful defiance of medical authority or a straightforward affirmation of a patient's right to die, but as a violent act. As Rebecca Garden points out, Justine ends Bessy's life "without discussing her plans directly with anyone, including Bessy." While Bessy does express a desire to die—"breathing out: 'I want to die'"[60]—Justine's final catalyst for administering morphine is Justine's own "inner voice."[61] As Garden notes, Justine's act of euthanasia ultimately "relieve[s] *herself*" of Bessy's suffering.[62]

It is therefore not wholly surprising that both John and Justine come to be haunted by Bessy's death and by their own perception that Dillon's life is expendable. In fact, through the thoughts of Justine and John, Wharton repeatedly brings Dillon's and Bessy's suffering into dialogue with each other, showing that they have both been marginalized by forms of care that truly amount to violence. Initially drawn to the mills' seeming vitality, John comes to feel trapped in a state of mind that is haunted by images of death following Justine's act of euthanasia: ". . . too often," he reflects, "one must still grope one's way through the personal difficulty by the dim taper carried in long-dead hands . . ."[63] Wharton's reference to "long-dead hands" recalls Dillon's injured hand, as ideas about Bessy's state and Dillon's perceived disposability merge into a single source of guilt and dread that threatens John's sense of vitality. A similar sense of imperiled vitality afflicts Justine as a nurse, who remains tormented by Bessy's death. From the outset, in her encounters with patients, Justine had lamented that it felt "cruel to be alive,"[64] in the face of so much suffering. After administering the lethal dose to Bessy, Justine questions her decision, describing how she feels mired in an atmosphere of illness and death: "she shook herself free from this morbid horror—the rebound of health was always prompt in her, and her mind instinctively rejected every form of moral poison . . ."[65] Here, the very phrase "moral poison" echoes Wharton's earlier description of the "morphia-poisoning" used to euthanize Bessy, underscoring the ethical ambiguity surrounding her act.[66] John and Justine both come to consider themselves as ensnared in a "web of tragic fatality"[67] as, although they attempt to forget Bessy's death, they remain traumatized by it. In the final scene, Bessy's memory appears as a "phantom" to be suppressed.[68] This resurfacing vocabulary of life, death, and vigor illustrates the hold that the act of euthanasia exerts on the characters' self-perception, relationships, and broader worldview.

While Bessy's death haunts John and Justine, their very attraction to each other becomes a cruelly twisted antidote to their morbid feelings. Their romance rejuvenates them. At one point, Justine is depicted as a "phoenix" rising from the ashes,[69] and Wharton writes that "there were moments when she was so mortally lonely that any sympathetic contact with another life sent a glow into her veins."[70] Like the "rush of life" that John experiences in the mills despite Dillon's injury, there is something perverse about this renewed sense of vitality that begins to emerge even as Bessy suffers. While Bessy is given a narcotic that ends her life after Justine recognizes that Bessy's love for John is itself already "dead,"[71] Justine continues to draw renewed energy and security from her relationship with John. At one point, with respect to her relationship with John, Wharton writes that Justine feels as though there is a "touch of a narcotic in her veins," a moment which creates an unsettling symmetry with the scene of the dose of a narcotic that is given to Bessy to end her life. Meanwhile, the continual renewal of John's energy through his relationship with Justine appears disturbing. Similarly to Bessy's state as she suffers, described as a kind of "half-life," John experiences a sense of partial life when he is away from Justine. While Justine at first worries over Bessy's paralyzed body that she would be relegated to a" desolate half-life which was the utmost that science could hold out,"[72] after Bessy's death, when Justine departs from John for some time, John realizes she has provided the "*vivifying* thought which gave meaning to the life he had chosen" as "his life was in truth one indivisible organism . . . Self and other-self were ingrown from the roots—whichever portion fate restricted him to would be but a mutilated *half-live* fragment of the whole" (emphasis my own).[73] Through this kind of parallelism, Wharton shows how Justine and John strive to sustain each other's compromised vitality in the wake of ongoing trauma and guilt.

Early reviewers, particularly those writing in medical venues, grappled with the medical ethics embedded in *The Fruit of the Tree* but not always with the specificities of disabled embodiment and experience that the novel foregrounded. A reviewer for the *Journal of the American Medical Association*, in an article titled "Euthanasia as a Romantic Motive," remarked that "no one who reads this book would ever care to have his own life shortened under such circumstances . . . After all, death impends more or less directly over all humanity, yet humanity finds some enjoyment in life for the time being."[74] In the *New York Medical Journal*, another critic disapproved of Wharton's depiction of a medical professional "knowingly administer[ing] a narcotic in a poisonous dose . . . to hasten the unavoidable end," calling it "murder in the most heinous form . . . taking advantage of the peculiar position of trust." This reviewer chastised Wharton for failing to punish Justine, as Justine does not appear to "suffer" enough from the recognition of her "wrongdoing."[75] Neither of these critiques recognized that Wharton eschewed a straightforward stance that would be universally applicable, complicating any effort to reduce her work to a single moral injunction applicable to all "humanity" or a commentary on the trustworthiness of the medical professions in general.

But while *Fruit* has the effect of refusing moral clarity, piercing through the novel's ambiguity is a critique of the specific ways disabled patients are often unfairly devalued. Wharton expressed a criticism of the way disability can become construed as marking patients as already dead or bound for an early death, and she also portrayed the able-bodied sustaining a sense of their own vitality by attempting to suppress the trauma produced by their encounters with debilitated patients and populations. Although from her correspondence it is clear that Wharton considered a right to die to be ethically tenable, the very complexity portrayed within *Fruit* about euthanasia reveals Wharton approaching physicians' increasing power over death with caution. By juxtaposing Justine and John's invigorating romance with their reductive assumption that disabled lives are disposable, Wharton pointed toward the need for physicians and nurses to remain vigilant and sensitive to disability, as she challenged pro-euthanasia arguments that risked both hastening patients' deaths and warping how it feels to be alive.

Against the Duty to Die

Later in the twentieth century, Hollywood screenwriter and fiction writer Dalton Trumbo's novel *Johnny Got His Gun* (1938) likewise explored the treatment of disability and euthanasia. As relayed in a *New York Times* article, Trumbo drew inspiration from two incidents involving disabled veterans of World War I. The first was a newspaper piece about the Prince of Wales, who remarked of a veteran in a Canadian military hospital: "The only way I could salute, the only way I could *communicate* with that man . . . was to kiss his cheek." The second was the account of a British major "so torn up that he was deliberately reported missing in action." It was only years later—after the soldier died in a military hospital—that this family learned the truth of his situation.[76]

Johnny Got His Gun fuses an anti-war message with a plea for better understanding disability through the character of a wounded, injured soldier. The novel was published shortly before World War Two, which Trumbo believed was "a moral war from our point of view, one that should be won." Although *Johnny Got His Gun* was initially intended as a critique of American interventionism in the First World War, Trumbo feared it might be dismissed as purely pacifist upon its release and tried to limit its readership. Nonetheless, the novel remained significant throughout the mid-twentieth century, particularly during the Vietnam War era. While its early reception centered on its anti-war perspective, Trumbo's message is equally committed to envisioning medical approaches free from ableism. Joe Bonham, the protagonist, is an American soldier critically injured by an artillery shell in World War I, left severely injured and, in a state of delirium and paralysis, unable to speak. Throughout, Trumbo intersperses Joe's reflections on the hospital environment with flashbacks to his pre-war life, merging the novel's pacifist concerns with a commentary on how disabled patients are perceived and treated. Although Joe's severe injuries may seem exceptional, Trumbo insisted they are more common than one might expect. In a 1968 letter regarding plans for a film adaptation, Trumbo refuted claims that his novel *Johnny Got His Gun* rested on a contrived "case history for which there is not one iota of proof outside the author's fevered imagination . . . the result of all possible exceptions—an exception so extreme that it verges on impossible," producing its "shock value." After its publication, he had encountered enough evidence—from his own experiences as a World War II correspondent as well as reports from a friend of severely injured Vietnam veterans—to confirm that these scenarios were real. In addition, he had heard from friends and the news about injured soldiers in Vietnam, and knew that "there are enormous hospitals all over the United States and Southeast Asia which are filled to capacity with wounded American soldiers," many of whom suffered in a way that was as "as bad as Joe, and conceivably worse."[77] Joe's injury is understood as an effect of a long history of US military intervention and debilitating social conditions more broadly.

In *Johnny Got His Gun*, Trumbo expresses a critical ambivalence about how the medical profession understands and cares for debilitated patients. On one level, Trumbo expresses recognition of the crucial importance of the medical professions in providing care. Joe recognizes the lifesaving skills of doctors and nurses: "The doctors were getting pretty smart especially now that they had three or four years in the army with plenty of raw material to experiment on. . . . If they got you quick enough. . . . they could save you from almost any kind of injury."[78] Similarly, Joe relies on the nurses both for medical treatment and for intimate companionship, as they hang his clothing and wash him. He understands one particular nurse as his genuine friend. Yet even as he depends on medical professionals, Joe articulates the need for them to understand disabled bodies and minds differently. He senses the physicians' tendency to reduce him to a spectacle: "the doctors who brought their friends in to see him would no longer say here is a man who has lived without arms legs ears eyes nose mouth isn't it wonderful?" and laments that "people were always willing to pay to see a curiosity... always interested in terrible sights," including himself.[79] Through Joe's perspective, Trumbo calls for the medical profession to recognize that disabled patients have complex interior lives, rather than viewing them as clinical marvels or reducing them to objects of pity.

As opposed to the way disability is often instrumentalized by the medical professions, Joe imagines strategically drawing attention to his disability to convey a social message about war's debilitating effects. Although Joe does not wish to be displayed as yet another medical spectacle, he imagines being exhibited as an "educational exhibit" in circuses and traveling carnivals, sealed in a glass coffin.[80] This vision underscores how the war has not only severely wounded him but has rendered him, according to how he perceives himself, already dead. Despite demanding professional medical care, Joe is wary of the medical professions' tendency to perceive his body as an object of morbid curiosity. Instead, he aims to make use of his disability to broadcast a politically charged critique of war's destructive power.

Yet the stigmatization of disability can shape not only the perspectives of physicians but also how patients perceive themselves. While Joe tries to transform his disability into a tool of anti-war advocacy, he also expresses internalized self-loathing assumptions about his own perceived uselessness. He worries that, if he were discharged from the hospital, "all his life... there would have to be people taking care of him," and because he has no money, "he would be a burden to people."[81] Even as he tries to wrest control of his body from this ableist logic, Joe's own fears reflect the tragic sense in which he has internalized the devaluation of his life.

Trumbo's critique focuses especially on the notion of a duty to die, which he suggests is both convoluted and senseless. Joe declares that no one should want to die for their country: "What the hell good to you is your native land after you're dead?... If you get killed fighting for your native land you've bought a pig in a poke."[82] Crucially, Trumbo insists that a right to die ought not to be conflated with the idea that disabled lives have no value. Joe resists any ideology that would demand that he die as a sacrifice for a cause. As Joe points out, the notion of death for a noble cause is absurd; once "you die... you've got no rights,"[83] and "only the dead know whether all these things people talk about are worth dying for or not..."[84] Any risk of one's life whether for national or other causes is presented as irrational, given the impossibility of knowing if the sacrifice is worthwhile.

In critiquing the duty to die through Joe's musings as a patient, Trumbo aligns his anti-war stance with a skepticism toward the same kind of logic that subtends pro-euthanasia arguments.

At the same time, Joe sometimes wishes to die—but keeping Trumbo's critique of the conventional treatment of disability in mind , particularly his repudiation of the duty to die, helps clarify Joe's own death wishes. Tethered to the hospital by tubes in his stomach, Joe likens these tubes to a womb, "except a baby in its mother's body could look forward to the time when it would live,"[85] inverting imagery of life with a reference to how he views himself as already dead. Viewing himself as "the nearest thing to a dead man on earth"[86] as justification for his thoughts about wanting to die, Joe's longing for death reflects the severity of his physical and psychological suffering, which is shared by countless injured veterans who "couldn't die no matter how hard they tried."[87] Critically, unlike Henry in Stephen Crane's "The Monster" or Dillon in Edith Wharton's *Fruit of the Tree*, it is Joe himself—not other characters—who views his own condition as being akin to death. In *Johnny*, Trumbo offers a rejection of a social imperative to die, even as he shows Joe personally experiencing a desire for death as release that stems from profound pain. Though Joe has internalized harmful social norms pertaining to disability he shields himself from any kind of perspective that would hold that his life lacks inherent value.

Trumbo resists any oversimplifications about Joe's ideas and questions about life and death, instead depicting them as layered with ambiguity and tension. A Warner Brothers production report on planning for ideas about a potential film adaptation of *Johnny Got His Gun* underscores this unsettling uncertainty, noting how in the novel Joe "gets rather frantic and says he wants to get out and goes on about all the things he wants to do . . . I can't quite make out whether he is meant to die then but I rather think so."[88] In the 1971 film version—ultimately produced outside the major studio system—through Morse code Joe explicitly begs for euthanasia from the medical staff, and a nurse attempts to comply before being stopped by her supervising doctor. Whereas the film version of *Johnny Got His Gun* stages a conflict over euthanasia among the medical staff while showing Joe unambiguously calling for assisted death, the novel adopts a more nuanced approach by describing Joe's own internal conflict in detail. Joe simultaneously wants medical help in ending his life and longs to survive. At one point, he pleads, "God give me rest take me away hide me let me die,"[89] yet these same ruminations about sleep and death appear alongside his pleasure in simply witnessing each dawn "every morning from now on."[90] Through free-associative reveries, his thoughts of rest and dying intermingle with flashes of ecstatic appreciation for wakefulness and life. Eventually, Joe entertains epic visions of a potential resurrection, imagining himself as "a new kind of Christ," as Trumbo transforms the religious imagery of martyrdom into a political plea for respect for debilitated patients and populations.[91] This imagined resurrection is not narrowly personal but instead extends to the "world of dead fathers and crippled brothers and crazy screaming sons," as Trumbo evokes a communal resurrection which he idealizes, in utopian terms, as a "perfect picture of the future."[92] While Joe might at first appear to be denied a future, in the realm of the imagination he has a jubilant fantasy of a "crippled" utopia that is characterized by injury, madness, and death, yet at the same time is imbued with ecstatic pleasure in life. As Trumbo resists the notion of an individual duty to die for the sake of a community, he embraces possibilities for collective survival.

In reflecting on his work in the late-1960's, Trumbo emphasized that *Johnny Got His Gun* and its film adaptation were fundamentally about life, not death. In letters to the film's producers, he objected to promotional language emphasizing the story's "terrifying" aspects or its "horror," insisting that his intentions had been misunderstood. Here, Trumbo confronted something akin to his character Joe's cynical notion that people will pay to see "terrible sights," as he faced pressures for the film to be marketed in ways that privileged the grotesque and macabre in order to attract an audience. Trumbo rejected the premise that *Johnny* was a particularly terrifying narrative. Far from creating a horror story about death, Trumbo wanted the work to be seen as a "love story"—depicting Joe's relationships with his girlfriend Kareen, his father, his mother, and the nurse who appears to share an intimate bond with him. Above all, though, Trumbo insisted *Johnny* was a celebration not only of romantic love but of "the love of life and respect for every living thing." "It is not a death-song," he wrote, distancing *Johnny Got His Gun* from a fixation on dying. Rather, he regarded the story as "a hymn of life."[93]

Trumbo continued to wrestle with the implications of having created a protagonist who at times wanted to die, but he emphasized above all Joe's consciousness of his own fundamental desire for life. He acknowledged the ethical complexities of physician-assisted death in the novel, while simultaneously underscoring Joe's will to live. "In connection with my deepest feeling that life must always oppose death and is always better than death (although death wins in the end)," Trumbo wrote as the film neared production, "I have discovered a curious thing about the novel and the screenplay . . . in both book and screenplay, Joe fights the injection of dope or sedatives. Why? If he were in pain, he would welcome it, wouldn't he?" Trumbo's answer was that the "only thing that really lives is [Joe's] mind," and if sedatives took that away, they would extinguish "all that remains of his life."[94] For this reason, once he realized this about his own novel, he scoured the film script to remove "all references to death as a release" until the very end, "that moment at the end when they tell him they cannot do the small thing which he asks." Only at that moment, Trumbo noted, "filled with such fury and despair as no one can imagine, he asks them for death."[95] Furthermore, even in the final moments of the film, where the request for euthanasia becomes explicit, Trumbo argued that, however paradoxically, Joe's call "is still, as it always was, to life,"[96] for in his understanding, he truly "asks not for death but for help."[97] He hoped that Joe's desire for life, much as was the case in the novel version of *Johnny* with Joe's dreams of collective resurrection, would spill over into a communal feeling of renewed vitality in the film's audience: "It will, I am sure, be impossible to erase from the audience's mind the extent of Joe's injuries, and the horror which resides in them (indeed, I would not want to erase them entirely), but I am determined that when the film ends, however stunned the audience may be by what it has seen, a good deal of the horror it feels at Joe's physical tragedy will be swamped by admiration for a fellow human who has done so much with so little; with an admiration for life and a desire to cling to it and live it; with, in short, admiration and respect for themselves because they are a *part* or [sic] life; with a feeling that they, who have so much more than Joe, have at least as good a reason to continue loving and living because life, any part of it that can function, is so infinitely better than death and the loss of love and loving and people."[98]

As *Johnny Got His Gun* and Trumbo's commentary reveal, early anxieties about euthanasia did not, by mid-century, resolve easily; they continued to unfold in evolving, increasingly nuanced ethical debates. In the post–World War II years, mainstream support for physician-assisted death in the United States gradually shifted away from the notion of a duty to die for a perceived social purpose toward an emphasis on personal rights, consent, and the individualized wishes of patients. Reflecting on *Johnny Got His Gun* later in the century, Trumbo continued to grapple with how he had represented a disabled character's death wishes. While *Johnny Got His Gun* remains ethically ambiguous with respect to the right to die, in Trumbo's portrayal and his understanding of his own work, a respect for disabled lives must become integral to modern medicine. While wrestling with the right to die, Trumbo exposed the absurdity of the notion of death as a duty. As he insisted, any conversation about physicians' newfound power over death could not be premised on notions that disabled patients' lives lacked inherent value.

In responding to evolving conversations about life, death, and disability, Edith Wharton, Stephen Crane, and Dalton Trumbo each mounted incisive critiques of the notion of the duty to die that shaped early twentieth-century debates on euthanasia. More specifically, they challenged the assumptions shaping modern medicine that were predicated on the view that disabled patients and populations were burdensome. Refusing to offer a neat set of medical-ethical directives, their fiction nevertheless unsettled any view that would reduce those in states of debility to being unworthy of life. These authors acknowledged that sometimes the desire to die can be an affirmation of individual autonomy, but that it must never be conflated with a broader cultural or institutional mandate of dying as a duty. Crane's portrayal of communally inflicted violence, Wharton's critique of industrial capitalism, and Trumbo's pacifism were all predicated on the recognition of the perils of slowly killing forms of debilitation. Within such conditions, as their fiction suggests, survival, lifesaving care, and the very commitment to valuing disabled patients' autonomy and lives become powerful forms of protest.

Coda

WHAT WOULD A PROGRESSIVE politics of professional medical care look like, and how has it been imagined? Some answers are provided by fiction writers who have both pointed to problems with the medical establishment and proposed solutions to health-related injustices. Robert Herrick, Wallace Thurman, A. L. Furman, and Frank Slaughter critiqued the capitalist economy of care while pointing toward possibilities for more affordable medical services. Charles Chesnutt, Walter White, and Ralph Ellison condemned entrenched medical racism and envisioned acts of medical care as forms of racial protest. Through their reform work and their novels on sexual health, Charlotte Perkins Gilman and Upton Sinclair challenged the pervasive culture of secrecy surrounding venereal disease; they also promoted strategies for claiming and reclaiming medical expertise to protect women's health. In critiquing the cultural logic of euthanasia that threatened medical professionalism, Edith Wharton, Stephen Crane, and Dalton Trumbo emphasized that doctors and nurses had a duty to respect and actively protect disabled lives. All of these authors paired challenges to the status quo within medicine with attempts at envisioning alternative forms of professional medical care and scientific expertise that could address them.

Since the origin of the field of the medical humanities, scholars and students operating within it have pointed to the necessity of cultivating a political approach to health and medicine that resonates with the central impulses behind these writers' fiction. The medical humanities emerged alongside and often drew from postwar movements for health justice, including, for instance, the Black Panther Party's establishment of community health programs beginning in the late 1960s;[1] the publication of *Our Bodies, Ourselves* by the Boston Women's Health Book Collective in 1970; the Young Lords' occupation of Lincoln Hospital in the South Bronx, New York City that same year; and the activism of the AIDS Coalition to Unleash Power in the late 1980s and early 1990s. As the medical humanities evolved, students began demanding an approach to health within their curricula that resonated with the energies animating countercultural protest movements. In 1984, physician and bioethicist Eric Cassell, in a Hastings Center report entitled

The Place of the Humanities in Medicine, reflected on these developments. Recounting the field's origins, he argued that the humanities—including the study of literary texts—should be employed to rehumanize medicine in an age of disenchantment. He observed that medical students were compelled to view the body "as a thing apart from and different from their own bodies," noting that "their cadavers, experimental physiology, pathology, indeed, all the preclinical studies provide a dehumanized arena in which to learn human biology." Cassell contended that physicians must undergo a process of "personalizing" in order to treat "whole persons," a process in which the humanities could play a crucial role. Yet while emphasizing this humanistic approach to medicine that privileged compassion and a consideration of the whole patient, he shifted from individual to social concerns when he noted that students were increasingly demanding that their medical humanities education address issues of poverty, racial bias, and oppression.[2] Cassell thought that science, as it applied to individual bodies, could be refined by the humanities, but he worried that students privileging countercultural protest were too quick to dismiss this authority of science. With time, Cassell argued, "it will become apparent again that science and technology are not the enemies; and there will be a more widespread understanding that 'reason' is not inherently atomistic or reductionist."[3] Because of this commitment to medical authority, Cassell had no patience for the "vast array of 'alternative therapies,' from acupuncture to Zen" as substitutes for "scientific medicine." These kinds of alternative therapies mirrored his view of students' political critiques of medical authority: both seemed to constitute misguided reversions to something akin to what Paul Starr refers to as the "therapeutic nihilism" of the nineteenth century, the notion that professional medicine was woefully ineffective and ought to be avoided entirely. He claimed that while these students were "clear-sighted" about the threat of medicine's complicity in political oppression, medical students of that generation "did not have a set of alternate concepts to put in place that *would be effective in the care of the sick.*"[4] He worried that medical students were attempting to dismantle conventional medical authority, but that they had nothing with which to replace it. For some early medical humanities scholars, commitments to health justice were threateningly anti-scientific and impractical. As Cassell rightly pointed out, "science and technology" did not have to be the "enemies," But as the writers I focus on in this book demonstrated, a commitment to health justice could in fact coexist with, and even become mutually co-constitutive of, a strategic recourse to medical facts, knowledge, and science.

While scholars and students in the health humanities have increasingly recognized the significance of centering health-justice concerns within the discussion of professional medicine in order to improve it, a parallel tradition in the late twentieth and early twenty-first centuries, appearing within the social sciences, literature, and cultural critique, has rejected conventional medicine. By the 1960s, the critique and even rejection of medical authority was becoming increasingly prominent. To be sure, these anti-medical arguments have posed significant challenges to complacency with an imperfect medical system. In *Medical Nemesis* (1974), Ivan Illich argued that twentieth-century professional medicine—with its sprawling bureaucracy, dehumanizing treatments, ineffective interventions, and scientific errors—had become a "major threat to health."[5] Although various strands of anti-medical thought have long been prevalent in the US, Illich's work represented a broader shift toward a resurgence of "therapeutic nihilism" around the mid to late twentieth century and continuing into the twenty-first century, emerging largely out of anti-psychiatric movements and also encompassing critiques of various aspects of professional medical care more generally, including attention to abuses of medical authority stemming from the perception of a fundamental power imbalance between physicians and patients. This kind of critique echoed in many ways the skepticism toward conventional medical authority that animated early American health reform before the professionalization of medical care at the turn of the century.[6]

Contemporary patients and writers who draw on lived experiences of physical and psychological suffering have been particularly critical of "the medical gaze,"[7] arguing that medical authorities often reductively oversimplify, dismiss, and misunderstand patients' histories and narratives. Many literary writers who explore the complex realities of illness and health have questioned the value of modern medicine altogether. For instance, in her 1997 essay "Gift of Disease," Kathy Acker probed the limits of the medical gaze as part of a broader critique of the medical-industrial complex's corruption of healing. She noted that "breast cancer, in the realm of Western medicine, is big business." Acker argued that modern medicine was entangled in a narrow framework of conventionality and normalcy, explaining: "My search for a way to defeat cancer now became a search for life and death that were meaningful. Not for the life presented by conventional medicine, a life in which one's meaning or self was totally dependent upon the words and actions of another person, even of a doctor. The hardest part of my cancer was walking away from that surgeon and from conventional medicine. Belief in conventional medicine, in what our doctors tell us, is so deeply ingrained in our society that to walk away from it is to walk away from normal society. Many of my friends phoned me, crying and yelling at me for not undergoing chemotherapy." Before her death, instead of relying on conventional professional medicine, Acker turned to alternative therapies, including "adjunctive cancer therapy," acupuncture, and the "Gerson method," a nutritional therapy discredited by the medical establishment. She recounts working in London with "an herbalist," "a cranial therapist," and the so-called "Barefoot Doctor," Stephen Russell, who sought to treat cancer by addressing patients' blockages of energy.[8] Acker's skepticism toward the medical profession compelled her to explore and document informal remedies as an act of resistance, before cancer claimed her life.

In the twenty-first century, continued experiences of violence, neglect, and inaccessibility within the medical establishment have fueled renewed skepticism toward medical science. In her memoir *The Undying* (2019), Anne Boyer articulates this skepticism: "There are . . . doctors who mislead people with benign or mild cancer-related conditions into aggressive, expensive treatment, or the doctors who do not tell patients they are dying, leading them into months of costly, painful, useless interventions."[9] Boyer critiques not only the profit-driven structures of health care but also the scientific legitimacy of contemporary treatments. She asserts that "many medical historians will view chemotherapy with the same perplexed curiosity that they once viewed formerly common practices such as bloodletting," which were often motivated by "superstition rather than science."[10] In Boyer's articulation, cancer treatment is characterized by uncertainty, deception, and a lack of effectiveness.

Owing to the kinds of failings in the medical system that these writers responded to, some prominent strands of critical work on health justice have increasingly turned to forms of care falling outside professional, institutional frameworks. As Lakshmi Piepzna-Samarasinha notes when discussing disability politics, health justice, and "care work," "people's fear of accessing care didn't come out of nowhere. It came out of generations and centuries in which needed care meant being locked up, losing your human and civil rights, and being subject to abuse."[11] For this reason, in imagining a revitalized politics of care, many advocates of health justice have looked beyond or turned away from the health care professions, privileging forms of informal care. As Akemi Nishida suggests, informal care is especially crucial in the twenty-first century, when social inequities in official health care have become deeply entrenched, and in this context, collective care can facilitate illness and disability justice. Confronted with a flawed and insufficient health care system, Nishida argues for the importance of a politics of care constituted by grassroots and mutual-aid groups. During the COVID-19 pandemic, forging health justice networks—through the collective dissemination of public health information, sharing resources such as food, masks, and hand sanitizer, and establishing supportive social media groups—proved vital.[12] In a similar vein, Johanna Hedva's seminal 2016 essay "Sick Woman Theory" draws on their personal experience with chronic illness to challenge the Western medical-insurance industrial complex. Hedva contends, "I am antagonistic to the notion that the Western medical-insurance industrial complex understands me in my entirety, though they seem to think they do." Hedva calls for a culture of interdependence and mutual support, suggesting that achieving health justice often requires direct interventions against institutional medical authority, as exemplified by their rejection of "the notion that one needs to be legitimated by an institution" in order for medical authorities to attempt to "fix you according to their terms."[13]

The principles animating these anti-medical critiques and endorsements of informal care emerge from deeply necessary and urgent commitments to health justice. At the same time, I have traced a distinct though in many ways complementary tradition of critique within the pages of American fiction of an earlier period, oriented toward grappling with how medicine, as a profession and institution, might itself be fixed. Authors have recognized that, so often, there are not viable alternatives to powerful institutions and systems of medicine. Though viewing modern medicine as either a source of harm or potential, they persistently centered possibilities for its transformation in their literary representations and in their politics.

Attending to fiction centering the conventional medical establishment remains essential, as many pressing health-related challenges require medical-professional solutions, such as expanded access to medical care, reforms in medical education, the accurate dissemination of public health information, and a commitment to addressing the concerns of chronically ill patients. Notably, the twenty-first century has witnessed a dangerous form of skepticism toward conventional medical authority, manifested in anti-mask politics, a willful disregard for scientific facts, the promotion of non-evidence-based remedies for COVID-19, and the dramatic cutting of funding to governmental health services. While, as Hedva argues, it is necessary to adopt a critical approach to modern medicine, it is equally important—especially in the face of resurgent, deeply regressive forms of therapeutic nihilism—to recognize how even established forms of medical authority can play a critical role in advancing health justice. Critics of medical authority rightly point to the dangers of moralistic, disciplinary, and consumerist medical attitudes toward health, but they still must often acknowledge the benefits of modern medicine. In a collection of essays arguing "against health," Jonathan Metzl asks rhetorically, "How can anyone take a stand against health? What could be wrong with health? Shouldn't we be for health?" In a polemical mode, Metzl critiques the ways that medical ideas seep into troubling and often stigmatizing cultural perceptions of bodies and minds. But even as Metzl critiques overly medicalized and harmful medical views of health, he notes that the contributors to the volume "believe in the germ theory of infectious illness" and in penicillin and "stand firmly behind recent expansions of healthcare coverage."[14] Especially in the contemporary moment, in which conventional notions of medical expertise are imperiled, it is imperative to consider how even the most pointed critiques of the medical establishment must often leave room for its expertise.

As part of the attempt to train generations of medical professionals in cultural competence and political engagement, health justice concerns have become increasingly recognized as critical for medical, pre-medical, and liberal arts education. A 2020 report from the Association of American Medical Colleges argued for "the fundamental role of the arts and humanities in medical education," noting that the first two decades of twenty-first-century medicine have witnessed significant transformations in healthcare delivery, pronounced health disparities, civil unrest, unprecedented rates of physician burnout and suicide, and unforeseen public health crises such as the opioid epidemic and the coronavirus pandemic. The report asserted that integrating the arts and humanities into medical education is essential to training a physician workforce capable of achieving optimal outcomes for patients and communities. Key benefits include enhanced professionalism and empathy but also "social advocacy."[15] More generally, the burgeoning field of the health humanities—as noted by Craig Klugman and Erin Lamb—is united by its commitment to "working explicitly toward social justice."[16]

This socially oriented critique of modern medicine does not negate the radical possibilities for self-care and alternative, less medicalized approaches to health; rather, this critique underscores how medical perspectives and lay wisdom can productively inform each other. To be sure, self-care has often been understood as a substitute for professional medicine. Kathy Acker, for example, described her engagement with the self as a means to demystify her diagnosis apart from the physician's authority, while Johanna Hedva conceptualized a powerful form of protest to entail not only caring for another but also for oneself—even in private, non-medical spaces. The contemporary concept of self-care emerges from Audre Lorde's work. While recovering from cancer and confronting a deeply flawed medical establishment—shaped by racism, sexism, ableism, and capitalism—Lorde argued in an oft-quoted passage from *A Burst of Light* (1988) that "caring for myself is not self-indulgence, it is self-preservation, and that is an act of political warfare."[17] In fact, this radical tradition of self-care can complement—rather than only unfold in opposition to—an embrace of medical authority. Jina B. Kim and Sami Schalk contend that "self-care is not . . . a rejection of medicine but, rather, an active and informed participation with medicine that recognizes the knowledge and insights of both patient and practitioner."[18] In a less-cited passage, Lorde noted that self-care "does not mean I give in to the belief, arrogant or naive, that I know everything I need to know in order to make informed decisions about my body." Instead, she maintained that "attending to my own health, gaining enough information to help me understand and participate in the decisions made about my body by people who know more medicine than I do, are crucial strategies in my battle for living."[19] In this view, in addition to self-care, cultivating a strategic dialogue with the medical profession is another kind of political warfare that demands to be waged.

The transformative reclamation of both self-care and professional medicine is particularly important in the twenty-first century, as the privatizing appropriation of self-care by medical industries threatens to exploit vulnerable populations. Although self-care has historically served as a form of political agency, it risks being co-opted by a deeply individualistic ideology. Hiʻilei Julia Kawehipuaakahaopulani Hobart and Tamara Kneese noted in 2020 that care had emerged as a crucial form of political empowerment. However, as they also suggest, digital health technologies, insurance discounts, and ideologies of self-health threaten to reduce self-care, in deeply unjust ways, to a profit-motivated bottom line: "... Self-care is thus popularly associated with self-optimization, or a way of preparing individuals for increased productivity in demanding workplaces when, in reality, things like chronic illness are incompatible with capitalist productivity and even visible forms of activism ..."[20] This ideology of self-care within modern medicine, combined with strains of wellness consumer culture that purport to empower individuals through a wide range of self-administered and alternative medicine products promoted via advertising and social media, detract attention from the need for collective resolutions to medical injustices.

Modern US fiction serves as a critical resource for understanding how professional medical authority might complement the democratizing potential of imaginative understandings of health that are rooted in traditions of social protest. In fact, this fiction frequently stages resonances between medical authority and transformative visions of patient autonomy. For example, consider the dialogue and alliance between Dr. William Miller and his patient Josh Green in Chesnutt's *The Marrow of Tradition*, the portrayal of Sylvia Castleman in Sinclair's *Sylvia's Marriage*, who takes charge of her health by consulting a medical bookstore, or the depiction of Henry Johnson's self-preservation in Crane's *The Monster*, which foreshadows Dr. Ned Trescott's life-saving care. In these instances, lay wisdom is effectively combined and entangled with an acknowledgment of the critical importance of medical expertise. More fundamentally, the very proliferation of US fiction with medical themes has contributed to health justice, combining a recourse to medical expertise with political perspectives that have privileged collectively held concerns. Since the origins of modern medicine, authors have challenged both therapeutic nihilism and a reductive optimism in medical progress, instead advocating for reconfigurations of who holds, represents, and wields medical authority, calling for improvements in the quality of professional medical care, and attending to the social causes and consequences of ill health. Like the patients they portrayed, who were necessarily reliant on the medical establishment for their care, they realized that it was precisely because of modern medicine's power to heal that it needed to be reformed and radically transformed.

Archival Collections

- Dalton Trumbo Papers. Special Collections at the University of California, Los Angeles.
- Dalton Trumbo Papers. Wisconsin Center for Film and Theater Research, University of Wisconsin–Madison.
- Edith Wharton Collection. Yale Collection of American Literature, Beinecke Rare Book and Manuscript Library.
- Frank Slaughter-Biographical Files. Rubenstein Library Archives, Duke University.
- John Ahouse-Upton Sinclair Collection, 1895–2014. California State University, Dominguez Hills.
- NAACP Papers. Library of Congress.
- Richard Wright Papers. Yale Collection of American Literature, Beinecke Rare Book and Manuscript Library.
- Ralph Ellison Papers. Manuscript Division, Library of Congress, Washington, DC.
- Robert Herrick Papers. Hanna Holborn Gray Special Collections Research Center, University of Chicago Library.
- Upton Sinclair Papers. Lilly Library, Indiana University.
- Upton Sinclair Collection. Albert and Shirley Small Special Collections Library, University of Virginia.

Notes

INTRODUCTION

1   Stephen J. Kunitz, "Professionalism and Social Control in the Progressive Era: The Case of the Flexner Report." *Social Problems* 22, no. 1 (1974).
2   Paul Starr, "The Politics of Therapeutic Nihilism," *The Hastings Center Report* 6, no. 5 (1976).
3   Nancy Tomes, *Remaking the American Patient: How Madison Avenue and Modern Medicine Turned Patients into Consumers* (University of North Carolina Press, 2016), 23.
4   John Tennent, *Every Man His Own Doctor; or, The Poor Planter's Physician* (Benjamin Franklin, 1734).
5   John C. Gunn, *Domestic Medicine; or, Poor Man's Friend* (1830).
6   Walt Whitman, *Manly Health and Training: To Teach the Science of a Sound and Beautiful Body* (Regan Arts, 2017).
7   James C. Whorton, *Crusaders for Fitness: The History of American Health Reformers* (1982; Princeton University Press, 2014).
8   Samuel Thomson, *New Guide to Health, or, Botanic family physician* (J. Howe, 1832).
9   Mary Sargeant Gove Nichols, *Mary Lyndon, Or Revelations of a Life; An Autobiography* (New York: W.A. Townsend and Company, 1855).
10 For discussions of the Civil War's pivotal role in expanding US hospitals and advancing medical science, see Shauna Devine, *Learning from the Wounded: The Civil War and the Rise of American Medical Science* (University of North Carolina Press, 2014). On the evolving image of American medical expertise, see Richard Malmsheimer, *Doctors Only: The Evolving Image of the American Physician* (Greenwood Press, 1988); and George B. Moseley III, "The US Health Care Non-System, 1908-2008," *AMA Journal of Ethics* 10, no. 5 (2008): 324–31. For an early perspective on the strides made by modern medicine, see William Osler, *The Evolution of Modern Medicine: A Series of Lectures Delivered at Yale University on the Silliman Foundation in April, 1913* (Yale University Press, 1921).
11 K. Patrick Ober, *Mark Twain and Medicine: "any Mummery Will Cure"* (University of Missouri Press, 2003).
12 *Mark Twain Speaking*, ed. Paul Fatout (University of Iowa Press, 1976).
13 *Mark Twain Speaking*, ed. Fatout.
14 William Carlos Williams, *The Autobiography of William Carlos Williams* (New Directions, 1967), 291.
15 Christopher R. Cashman, "Golden Ages and Silver Screens: The Construction of the Physician Hero in 1930–1940 American Cinema," *Journal of Medical Humanities* 40, no. 4 (2019).
16 On the contested notion of a golden age of medicine, see Allan M. Brandt and Martha Gardner, "The Golden Age of Medicine?" in *Companion to Medicine in the Twentieth Century*, ed. Roger Cooter and John Pickstone (Routledge, 2003), John C.

Burnham, "American Medicine's Golden Age: What Happened to It?" *Science*, 215, no. 4539, (1982); and Bert Hansen, *Picturing Medical Progress from Pasteur to Polio: A History of Mass Media Images and Popular Attitudes in America* (Rutgers University Press, 2009).

17 Joan Burbick, *Healing the Republic: The Language of Health and the Culture of Nationalism in Nineteenth-Century America* (Cambridge University Press, 1994). Josh Doty, *The Perfecting of Nature: Reforming Bodies in Antebellum Literature* (University of North Carolina Press, 2020), 9.

18 Susan Sontag, *Illness as Metaphor and AIDS and Its Metaphors* (Picador, 2013) [1978, 1989].

19 Sander L. Gilman, *Disease and Representation: Images of Illness from Madness to AIDS* (Cornell University Press, 1988), 9–10.

20 Lawrence Rothfield, *Vital Signs: Medical Realism and Nineteenth-Century Fiction* (Princeton University Press, 1992), xiv.

21 Amanda Claybaugh, *The Novel of Social Purpose: Literature and Social Reform in the Anglo-American World* (Cornell University Press, 2007).

22 Arthur Frank, *The Wounded Storyteller: Body, Illness, and Ethics* (University of Chicago Press, 1995); Rita Charon, *Narrative Medicine: Honoring the Stories of Illness* (Oxford University Press, 2006), viii; Sari Altschuler, *The Medical Imagination: Literature and Health in the Early United States* (University of Pennsylvania Press, 2018).

23 For examples of literary criticism on medical professionalism on this period, see Cynthia Davis, *Bodily and Narrative Forms: The Influence of Medicine on American Literature, 1845–1915* (Stanford University Press, 2000); Lilian R. Furst, *Between Doctors and Patients: The Changing Balance of Power* (University of Virginia Press, 1998); Stephanie Browner, *Profound Science and Elegant Literature: Imagining Doctors in Nineteenth-Century America* (University of Pennsylvania Press, 2005).

CHAPTER ONE

1 Raymond Chandler, "It's All Right—He Only Died," *Strand Magazine*, October–February 2017, 6–7.

2 Matthew Haag, "Unearthed Raymond Chandler Story Rebukes US Health Care System," *The New York Times*, November 22, 2017.

3 Florence Greenberg, "A Spokeswoman for Workers' Families," The Nation's Health, Interdepartmental Committee to Coordinate Health and Welfare Activities, US Government Printing Office, Proceedings of the National Health Conference (Washington, DC, July 1938): 84.

4 Michael R. Grey, *New Deal Medicine: The Rural Health Programs of the Farm Security Administration* (Johns Hopkins University Press, 1999).

5 Rebecca Harding Davis, "Life in the Iron Mills," *Atlantic Monthly* 7, no. 42 (1861).

6 Edward Bellamy, *Looking Backward: 2000–1887*, ed. Alex MacDonald (Broadview Press, 2003), 114.

7 William Carlos Williams, *The Doctor Stories*, ed. Robert Coles (New Directions, 1984), 96.

8 James Rorty, *American Medicine Mobilizes* (W.W. Norton & Company, 1939), 15.

9 Phillip Barrish, "The Sticky Web of Medical Professionalism: Robert Herrick's *The Web of Life* and the Political Economy of Health Care at the Turn of the Century," *American Literature* 86, no. 3 (2014).

10 Herrick, *The Healer*, 38.
11 Herrick, *The Healer*, 40.
12 Hildegard Hoeller suggests that gifts are integral to US fiction as "vehicles that allow writers to tell stories about capitalism while . . . they also bring those narratives to the brink of reason and reveal their aporias." Hildegard Hoeller, "Capitalism, Fiction, and the Inevitable, (Im)Possible, Maddening Importance of the Gift," *PMLA* 127, no. 1 (2012): 132. One crucial earlier discussion of the role of the "gift" in modernity is to be found in the work of Marcel Mauss. Marcel Mauss, *The Gift: The Form and Reason for Exchange in Archaic Societies* (1925; Routledge, 2002).
13 Herrick, *The Healer*, 138–39.
14 Herrick, *The Healer*, 144.
15 Herrick, *The Healer*, 143.
16 Leo Marx, *The Machine in the Garden: Technology and the Pastoral Ideal in America* (Oxford University Press, 1964).
17 Cutting from *The Yorkshire Post*, January 24, 1912, box 23, folder 2, The Robert Herrick Papers, University of Chicago Library.
18 William R. Higgins, "David Graham Phillips, Robert Herrick and the Doctor: A Turn of the Century Dilemma," *American Transcendental Quarterly* 2, no. 2 (1988).
19 Herrick, *The Healer*, 312–13.
20 Herrick, *The Healer*, 334.
21 Herrick, *The Healer*, 335.
22 Blake Nevius, *Robert Herrick: The Development of a Novelist* (University California Press, 1962), 114–15.
23 Herrick, *The Healer*, 406.
24 Herrick, *The Healer*, 425.
25 Herrick, *The Healer*, 418.
26 Herrick, *The Healer*, 420.
27 Herrick, *The Healer*, 419.
28 Cutting from *The Colne Valley Guardian*, March 3, 1912, box 23, folder 22, The Robert Herrick Papers, University of Chicago Library.
29 Herrick, *The Healer*, 455.
30 Clipping, 1912, box 23 folder 2, The Robert Herrick Papers, University of Chicago Library.
31 "The Healer," *JAMA* 58, no. 1 (1912): 56–7.
32 "Dr. L.F. Barker in Novel: Friends Recognize Him in Robert Herrick's *The Healer*," *The Baltimore Sun*, December 24, 1911.
33 Wallace Thurman, "Autobiographical Statement," in *The Collected Writings of Wallace Thurman*, ed. by Amritjit Singh and Daniel M. Scott III (Rutgers University Press, 2003), 92.
34 Wallace Thurman, "Letters to Langston Hughes," in *The Collected Writings of Wallace Thurman*, ed. by Amritjit Singh and Daniel M. Scott III (Rutgers University Press, 2003), 131.
35 Sandra Opdyke, *No One Was Turned Away: The Role of Public Hospitals in New York City Since 1900* (Oxford University Press, 1999), 44.
36 Thurman and Furman, *The Interne*, 228–29.
37 Harry Hansen, "'The Interne' is Sensational But Ineffective Work: Aims to Expose Hospital 'Racket,' But Fails as a Novel," *The Minneapolis Sunday Tribune*, May 29, 1932.

38 Geoffrey Terwilliger, "Some of the Most Recent Spring Fiction: Hospital Racket," *New York Herald Tribune*, May 15, 1932.
39 Wallace Thurman and Abraham L. Furman, *The Interne* (The Macaulay Company, 1932), 33.
40 Thurman and Furman, *The Interne*, 68.
41 Thurman and Furman, *The Interne*, 114.
42 Thurman and Furman, *The Interne*, 46.
43 Thurman and Furman, *The Interne*, 31–32.
44 Mary Ziegler, *Dollars for Life: The Anti-abortion Movement and the Fall of the Republican Establishment* (Yale University Press, 2022), 2.
45 Leslie J. Reagan, *When Abortion Was a Crime: Women, Medicine, and the Law in the United States, 1867–1973* (University of California Press, 1997).
46 Karen Weingarten, *Abortion in the American Imagination* (Rutgers University Press, 2014).
47 Thurman and Furman, *The Interne*, 219.
48 Thurman and Furman, *The Interne*, 240.
49 Thurman and Furman, *The Interne*, 247.
50 Lee Edelman, *No Future: Queer Theory and the Death Drive* (Duke University Press, 2004).
51 Thurman and Furman, *The Interne*, 250.
52 Thurman and Furman, *The Interne*, 249.
53 Thurman and Furman, *The Interne*, 249–50.
54 "Frank G. Slaughter," Publicity Department, Doubleday & Company (New York: 1967), Box 23, Frank Slaughter Papers, Duke University Libraries.
55 Mary Ellen Wolcott, "Medicine, Writing Mix for Dr. Slaughter," *Asheville Citizen*, October 5, 1972.
56 "Frank G. Slaughter," From: Publicity Department, Doubleday & Company (New York: 1967)," box 23, Frank Slaughter Papers, Duke University Libraries.
57 Mary Ellen Wolcott, "Medicine, Writing Mix For Dr. Slaughter," *Asheville Citizen*, Oct. 5, 1972.
58 Frank Slaughter, "When the Scalpel Sharpens the Pen," *JAMA* 200, no. 1 (1967): 127.
59 Frank Slaughter, *That None Should Die* (The Book League of America, 1941), 94.
60 Slaughter, *That None Should Die*, 99.
61 Slaughter, *That None Should Die*, 112.
62 Jacqueline H. Wolf, *Cesarean Section: An American History of Risk, Technology, and Consequence* (Johns Hopkins University Press, 2020).
63 Slaughter, *That None Should Die*, 149–50.
64 Slaughter, *That None Should Die*, 150.
65 Beatrix Hoffman, *Health Care for Some: Rights and Rationing in the United States since 1930* (University of Chicago Press, 2012), xx.
66 Slaughter, *That None Should Die*, 384.
67 Slaughter, *That None Should Die*, 269.
68 See Lauren Berlant's discussion of the "humanizing" emotions. Lauren Berlant, *Compassion: The Culture and Politics of an Emotion* (Routledge, 2004).
69 Slaughter, *That None Should Die*, 303.
70 Slaughter, *That None Should Die*, 324.

71 John Warner, "The Fielding H. Garrison Lecture: The Aesthetic Grounding of Modern Medicine," *Bulletin of the History of Medicine* 88, no. 1 (2014): 4.
72 Jill Lepore, "The Lie Factory," *The New Yorker*, September 17, 2012.
73 Wolcott, "Medicine, Writing Mix."
74 Slaughter, *That None Should Die*, 166.
75 Economist Kenneth Arrow would observe in 1963 that despite intense debates over government involvement, charitable hospitals have persisted in the US precisely because of a tradition that embraces "human rights to adequate medical care," as evidenced by the "overwhelming predominance of nonprofit over proprietary hospitals." Kenneth Arrow "Uncertainty and the Welfare Economics of Medical Care," *The American Economic Review* 53, no. 5 (1963), 950.
76 Slaughter, *That None Should Die*, 257.
77 Slaughter, *That None Should Die*, 422.
78 Slaughter, *That None Should Die*, 422.
79 Slaughter, *That None Should Die*, 422–23.
80 Slaughter, *That None Should Die*, 317.
81 Arnold S. Relman, "The New Medical-Industrial Complex," *New England Journal of Medicine* 303, no. 17 (1980).
82 Frank Slaughter, "When the Scalpel Sharpens the Pen," *JAMA* 200, no. 1 (1967):126.
83 Frank Slaughter, "A Functional Model for Improving the Medical Care System," *Bulletin of The New York Academy of Medicine*, 49, no. 5 (1973), 367.
84 Slaughter, "Functional Model," 366.
85 Slaughter, "Functional Model," 366–7.
86 Slaughter, "Functional Model," 368.
87 Slaughter, "Functional Model," 364–5.
88 Slaughter, "Functional Model," 368.
89 Calvin Plimpton, "Discussion of Paper by Frank G. Slaughter, M.D.: A Functional Model for Improving the Medical Care System," *Bulletin of the New York Academy of Medicine*, 49, no. 5 (1973).
90 "Interview with Dr. Frank Slaughter, author, Fall 1973," *Radio TV Services Records*, circa 1937–2012," box 12, Duke University Libraries.

CHAPTER TWO

1 Marita Bonner, "Drab Rambles," in *Frye Street & Environs: The Collected Works of Marita Bonner*, ed. Joyce Flynn and Joyce Occomy Stricklin (Beacon Press, 1987), 93.
2 Bonner, "Drab Rambles," 97.
3 Bonner, "Drab Rambles," 97.
4 As Britt Rusert has shown, nineteenth-century African American literature and cultural expression often critiqued racial science. Although a widening separation between literature and science emerged at the turn of the twentieth century, as literature and science both became more professionalized, the twentieth century continued to witness literary critiques of racial bias in scientific medicine. Britt Rusert, *Fugitive Science: Empiricism and Freedom in Early African American Culture* (New York University Press, 2017), 222.
5 Thomas J. Ward, *Black Physicians in the Jim Crow South* (University of Arkansas Press, 2003).

6   Abraham Flexner and Henry S. Pritchett, M*edical Education in the United States and Canada; a Report to the Carnegie Foundation for the Advancement of Teaching*, Bulletin No. 4 (New York City, 1910), 180.
7   Charles Waddell Chesnutt, *Charles W. Chesnutt : Essays and Speeches*, ed. Joseph R. McElrath, Jr., Robert C. Leitz, III, and Jesse S. Crisler (Stanford University Press, 1999).
8   Vanessa Northington Gamble, *Making a Place for Ourselves: The Black Hospital Movement, 1920–1945* (Oxford University Press, 1995), 11.
9   Charles W. Chesnutt, "The Ideal Nurse," 372.
10 Chesnutt, "The Ideal Nurse," 377.
11 Chesnutt, "The Ideal Nurse," 377.
12 Chesnutt, "The Ideal Nurse," 377.
13 Chesnutt, "The Ideal Nurse," 389.
14 Chesnutt, "The Ideal Nurse," 380–81.
15 Chesnutt, "The Ideal Nurse," 381.
16 Chesnutt, "The Ideal Nurse," 381.
17 Chesnutt, "The Ideal Nurse," 381.
18 Chesnutt, "The Ideal Nurse," 381.
19 Chesnutt, "The Ideal Nurse," 380.
20 Chesnutt, "The Ideal Nurse," 380.
21 Chesnutt, "The Ideal Nurse," 381.
22 Helen M Chesnutt, *Charles Waddell Chesnutt, Pioneer of the Color Line* (University of North Carolina Press, 1952).
23 Charles W. Chesnutt to Booker T. Washington, July 21, 1910, *The Charles W. Chesnutt Archive*, edited by Stephanie P. Browner, Matt Cohen, and Kenneth M. Price.
24 Helen M. Chesnutt, *Charles Waddell Chesnutt, Pioneer of the Color Line* (University of North Carolina Press, 1952), 380.
25 Stephanie P. Browner, *Profound Science and Elegant Literature: Imagining Doctors in Nineteenth-Century America* (University of Pennsylvania Press, 2005), 210.
26 Susan Danielson, "Charles Chesnutt's Dilemma: Professional Ethics, Social Justice, and Domestic Feminism in *The Marrow of Tradition*," *Southern Literary Journal* 41 (Fall 2008), 76.
27 Brian Sweeney, "Doctor Jekyll and Mister Jim Crow: Medical Professionalism, Race, and Postsentimentalism in *The Marrow of Tradition*," in *The Sentimental Mode: Essays in Literature, Film and Television*, ed. Jennifer A Williamson, Jennifer Larson, and Ashley Reed (McFarland, 2014), 18.
28 Charles W. Chesnutt, *The Marrow of Tradition* (Houghton Mifflin, 1901), 283.
29 Kevin Kelly Gaines, *Uplifting the Race: Black Leadership, Politics, and Culture in the Twentieth Century* (University of North Carolina Press, 1996), 2.
30 Stephen P. Knadler, *Vitality Politics: Health, Debility, and the Limits of Black Emancipation* (University of Michigan Press, 2019).
31 Andreá N. Williams, *Dividing Lines: Class Anxiety and Postbellum Black Fiction* (University of Michigan Press, 2013).
32 Chesnutt, *The Marrow of Tradition*, 68.
33 Chesnutt, *The Marrow of Tradition*, 71–72.
34 Chesnutt, *The Marrow of Tradition*, 71.
35 Chesnutt, *The Marrow of Tradition*, 112.

36 Chesnutt, *The Marrow of Tradition*, 114.
37 Chesnutt, *The Marrow of Tradition*, 295.
38 Chesnutt, *The Marrow of Tradition*, 112.
39 Chesnutt, *The Marrow of Tradition*, 114.
40 Chesnutt, *The Marrow of Tradition*, 309.
41 William Gleason, "Voices at the Nadir: Charles Chesnutt and David Bryant Fulton," *American Literary Realism, 1870–1910* 24, no. 3 (1992): 32.
42 Chesnutt, *The Marrow of Tradition*, 315
43 Chesnutt, *The Marrow of Tradition*, 289.
44 Chesnutt, *The Marrow of Tradition*, 296.
45 Chesnutt, *The Marrow of Tradition*, 297
46 Chesnutt, *The Marrow of Tradition*, 65.
47 Chesnutt, *The Marrow of Tradition*, 65.
48 Chesnutt, *The Marrow of Tradition*, 64.
49 Chesnutt, *The Marrow of Tradition*, 65.
50 Chesnutt, *Marrow of Tradition*, 318.
51 Walter White, "Sept. 4, 1934," Papers of the NAACP, Library of Congress, 3.
52 Walter White, "Sept. 4, 1934," 4.
53 Walter White, "Sept. 4, 1934," 6.
54 Walter White, "The Negro Renaissance (1926)," in *The New Negro: Readings on Race, Representation, and African American Culture, 1892–1938*, ed. Henry Louis Gates, Jr., and Gene Andrew Jarrett (Princeton University Press, 2007), 353.
55 Walter White, *The Fire in the Flint* (Knopf, 1924), 11.
56 White, *The Fire in the Flint*, 12.
57 White, *The Fire in the Flint*, 24.
58 White, *The Fire in the Flint*, 65.
59 White, *The Fire in the Flint*, 139.
60 White, *The Fire in the Flint*, 98.
61 White, *The Fire in the Flint*, 188.
62 William Edward Burghardt Du Bois, *The Philadelphia Negro: A Social Study* (University of Pennsylvania, 1899), 113.
63 White, *The Fire in the Flint*, 48.
64 White, *The Fire in the Flint*, 48.
65 White, *The Fire in the Flint*, 57.
66 White, *The Fire in the Flint*, 58.
67 White, *The Fire in the Flint*, 226.
68 White, *The Fire in the Flint*, 289.
69 White, *The Fire in the Flint*, 290.
70 White, *The Fire in the Flint*, 11.
71 White, *The Fire in the Flint*, 236.
72 Walter White to Pennsylvania Medical Society, October 21, 1936, Southern Medical Society, Papers of the NAACP, Library of Congress.
73 Walter White, "'Negro Medical Ghetto' Exposed in Article by Howard Professor" *New York Herald Tribune* (August 24, 1947), A8.
74 United States Congress Senate Committee on Labor and Public Welfare, Veterans' Hospital Program: Hearings, Eightieth Congress, Second Session, on H. Con. Res. 54. and S. 1414. February 2, 3, 6, and 10, 1948 (US Government Printing Office, 1948).

75. US Congress Senate Committee on Labor and Public Welfare, 91.
76. US Congress Senate Committee on Labor and Public Welfare, 111.
77. "Negro V.A. Hospital is Rejected in House," *The New York Times*, June 7, 1951.
78. Walter White, *A Man Called White: The Autobiography of Walter White* (Viking, 1948), 63.
79. White, *A Man Called White*, 63–4.
80. White, *A Man Called White*, 64.
81. Walter White, "A Worthy Man of Science Gets a Tribute that is Well Deserved," *Chicago Defender* (April 12, 1952), 11.
82. *No Way Out*, directed by Joseph Mankiewicz, (1950; USA: Twentieth Century Fox).
83. Walter White, "'No Way Out' A Picture Scarcely without Equal," *Chicago Defender*, August 26, 1950, 7.
84. Joel Braslow, *Mental Ills and Bodily Cures: Psychiatric Treatment in the First Half of the Twentieth Century* (University of California Press, 1997).
85. Samuel Cartwright, "Report on the Diseases and Physical Peculiarities of the Negro Race," *New Orleans Medical and Surgical Journal* 7 (May 1851), 707.
86. Arrah B. Evarts, "Dementia Precox in the Colored Race," *The Psychoanalytic Review* 1 (1913), 394.
87. Robert Bendiner, "Psychiatry Comes to Harlem," *Negro Digest* 6, no. 11 (Summer 1948), 81.
88. Gabriel N. Mendes, *Under the Strain of Color: Harlem's Lafargue Clinic and the Promise of Antiracist Psychiatry* (Cornell University Press, 2015).
89. James E. Reibman, "Ralph Ellison, Frederic Wertham, M.D., and the Lafargue Clinic: Civil Rights and Psychiatric Services in Harlem," *Oklahoma City University Law Review* 26, no. 3 (2001).
90. Shelly Eversley. "The Lunatic's Fancy and the Work of Art." *American Literary History* 13, no. 3 (2001), 456.
91. J. Bradford Campbell, "The Schizophrenic Solution: Dialectics of Neurosis and Anti-Psychiatric Animus in Ralph Ellison's Invisible Man," *Novel* 43, no. 3 (2010), 460–61.
92. Cera Smith, "Shocking Therapy: Narrating Racism's Psychobiological Injuries in Ralph Ellison's Factory Hospital," *American Literature* 96, no. 3 (2024).
93. La Marr Jurelle Bruce, *How to Go Mad without Losing Your Mind: Madness and Black Radical Creativity* (Duke University Press, 2021), 25.
94. Ralph Ellison, "Beating that Boy," in *Shadow and Act*, (Vintage Books, 1964), 100.
95. Ellison, "Richard Wright's Blues," in *Shadow and Act*, 90.
96. Ellison, "Richard Wright's Blues," 92.
97. Ellison, "Harlem Is Nowhere," *Harper's* (August 1964).
98. Ellison, "Harlem Is Nowhere," (1947–1948), Box 1: 100, Ralph Ellison Papers, Library of Congress.
99. Ellison, "Harlem Is Nowhere" (1947–1948), Ralph Ellison Papers.
100. Ellison, "Harlem Is Nowhere" (1947–1948), Ralph Ellison Papers.
101. Ellison, "Harlem Is Nowhere" (1947–1948), Ralph Ellison Papers.
102. Ellison, "Harlem Is Nowhere" (1947–1948), Ralph Ellison Papers.
103. Ellison, "The Shadow and the Act," in *Shadow and Act*, 278.
104. Ellison, "The Shadow and the Act," 278.

105 Badia Sahar Ahad, *Freud Upside Down: African American Literature and Psychoanalytic Culture* (University of Illinois Press, 2010).
106 Ralph Ellison, *Invisible Man* (Vintage, 1995), 14.
107 Anne Anlin Cheng, *The Melancholy of Race: Psychoanalysis, Assimilation, and Hidden Grief* (Oxford University Press, 2001), 127.
108 Ellison, *Invisible Man*, 86.
109 Ellison, *Invisible Man*, 93.
110 Ellison, *Invisible Man*, 87.
111 Ellison, *Invisible Man*, 92.
112 Jonathan Metzl, *The Protest Psychosis: How Schizophrenia Became a Black Disease* (Beacon Press, 2010).
113 Walter Bromberg and Franck Simon, "The 'Protest' Psychosis," *Archives of General Psychiatry* 19, no. 2 (1968): 155.
114 Students of Karpman, "Psychological studies of Native Son, typescripts, corrected/1940," Box 90, folders 1108–1110, Series I: Writings of Others, Richard Wright Papers, Yale Collection of American Literature, Beinecke Rare Book and Manuscript Library.
115 William H. Grier and Price M. Cobbs, *Black Rage* (1968; Basic Books, 1980), 4.
116 Grier and Cobbs, *Black Rage*, 10.
117 Ellison, *Invisible Man*, 14.
118 Ellison, *Invisible Man*, 93.
119 Ellison, *Invisible Man*, 95.
120 Ellison, *Invisible Man*, 93.
121 Bendiner, "Psychiatry Comes to Harlem," 81.
122 Ellison, "Harlem is Nowhere," *Shadow and Act*.
123 Ellison, *Invisible Man*, 85.
124 Grier and Cobbs, *Black Rage*, 12.
125 Calvin C. Hernton, *Scarecrow* (Doubleday, 1974).
126 Michel Oren, "The Enigmatic Career of Hernton's 'Scarecrow,'" *Callaloo* 29, no. 2 (2006)
127 Ellison, *Invisible Man*, 231.
128 Ellison, *Invisible Man*, 233.
129 Ellison, *Invisible Man*, 236.
130 Ellison, *Invisible Man*, 236.
131 Ellison, *Invisible Man*, 238.
132 Ellison, *Invisible Man*, 238.
133 Ellison, *Invisible Man*, 240.
134 Ellison, *Invisible Man*, 237.
135 Ellison, *Invisible Man*, 233.
136 Ellison, *Invisible Man*, 242.
137 Ann Folwell Stanford, *Bodies in a Broken World: Women Novelists of Color and the Politics of Medicine* (University of North Carolina Press, 2003), 17.
138 Martha Cutter, "When Black Lives Really Do Matter: Subverting Medical Racism through African-Diasporic Healing Rituals in Toni Morrison's Fiction," *MELUS* 46, no. 4 (Winter 2021).

CHAPTER THREE

1 Annie Nathan Meyer, *It's Been Fun: An Autobiography* (Henry Schuman, 1951), 218.
2 I use the outdated term "venereal disease" as it was used in the period of composition of the texts I analyze in this chapter.
3 Annie Nathan Meyer, *Helen Brent, MD* (Cassell Publishing Company, 1892), 71.
4 Meyer, *It's Been Fun*, 218.
5 James Oppenheim, *Wild Oats* (B.W. Huebsch, 1910), 134.
6 Oppenheim, *Wild Oats*, 134.
7 Oppenheim, *Wild Oats*, 136.
8 Oppenheim, *Wild Oats*, 187.
9 Oppenheim, *Wild Oats*, 195.
10 Oppenheim, *Wild Oats*, 260.
11 42nd Congress, 3rd session, Senate of the United States (1873), "A Bill for the Suppression of Trade in, and Circulation of, obscene Literature and Articles of Immoral Use."
12 Scott Stern, *The Trials of Nina McCall* (Beacon Press, 2018).
13 Prince A. Morrow, *Social Diseases and Marriage: Social Prophylaxis* (Lea Bros., 1904), 22.
14 Prince A. Morrow, "The Problem of Social Hygiene," *The Medical Times* (June 1909), 166.
15 Stephanie Peebles Tavera, *(P)rescription Narratives: Feminist Medical Fiction and the Failure of American Censorship* (Edinburgh University Press, 2022).
16 Charlotte Perkins Gilman, *The Crux* (Charlton Company, 1911), 5.
17 Charlotte Perkins Gilman, "Comment and Review," *The Forerunner* 1 no. 6 (1910), 23.
18 William J. Robinson, *Never-Told Tales* (The Altrurians, 1910), 13.
19 Robinson, *Never-Told Tales*, 17.
20 Catherine Beecher, *A Treatise on Domestic Economy, Revised Edition* (Harper and Bros, 1848).
21 Gilman, "Kitchen-Mindedness," *The Forerunner*, 1, no. 4 (1910), 10–11.
22 Gilman, *Women and Economics: A Study of the Economic Relation Between Men and Women as a Factor in Social Evolution* (Small, Maynard & Company, 1898), 169.
23 Gilman, *Women and Economics*, 238.
24 Gilman, "Comment and Review," 1 no. 6, 22.
25 Gilman, "Comment and Review," 1 no. 6, 22.
26 Lavinia Dock, *Hygiene and morality; a manual for nurses and others, giving an outline of the medical, social, and legal aspects of the venereal diseases* (G.P. Putnam's Sons, 1910), 136.
27 Prince A. Morrow, *Social Diseases and Marriage: Social Prophylaxis* (Lea Bros., 1904), 182.
28 Morrow, *Social Diseases and Marriage*, 31.
29 Louise Newman, *White Women's Rights: The Racial Origins of Feminism in the United States* (Oxford University Press, 1999); Dana Seitler, "Unnatural Selection:

Mothers, Eugenic Feminism, and Charlotte Perkins Gilman's Regeneration Narratives," *American Quarterly* 55, no. 1 (2003); Ewa Luczak, *Breeding and Eugenics in the American Literary Imagination: Heredity Rules in the Twentieth Century* (Palgrave Macmillan, 2015).

30 Linda Gordon. *Woman's Body, Woman's Right: Birth Control in America: A Social History of Birth Control in America* (Viking, 1976), 134.
31 Mary Ziegler, "Eugenic Feminism: Mental Hygiene, the Women's Movement, and the Campaign for Eugenic Legal Reform, 1900-1935," *Harvard Journal Law and Gender* 211 (2008).
32 Gilman, "Should a Medical Certificate of Freedom from Transmissible Disease be Required as a Condition of License to Marry—III. In Its Sociological Aspects," *Transactions of the American Society of Sanitary and Moral Prophylaxis* 3 (1910), 143.
33 Charlotte Perkins Gilman, *The Crux* (Charlton Company, 1911), 221.
34 Gilman, *The Crux*, 212-13.
35 Gilman, *The Crux*, 219.
36 Gilman, *The Crux*, 225.
37 Gilman, *The Crux*, 245.
38 Cynthia J. Davis, *Charlotte Perkins Gilman: A Biography* (Stanford University Press, 2010), 63.
39 Charlotte Perkins Gilman, *The Living of Charlotte Perkins Gilman: An Autobiography* (University of Wisconsin Press, 1990 [1935]), 83.
40 Cindy Weinstein, *Family, Kinship, and Sympathy in Nineteenth-Century American Literature* (Cambridge University Press, 2004), 9.
41 Allan M. Brandt, *No Magic Bullet: A Social History of Venereal Disease in the United States* (Oxford University Press, 1985), 17.
42 Morrow, *Social Diseases and Marriage*, 61.
43 Gilman, *The Crux*, 210.
44 Gilman, *The Crux*, 211.
45 Gilman, *The Crux*, 212.
46 Victoria Woodhull, "The Elixir of Life: or, Why Do We Die? An Oration," in *Selected Writings of Victoria Woodhull: Suffrage, Free Love, and Eugenics*, ed. Cari M. Carpenter (University of Nebraska Press, 2010), 186.
47 Woodhull, "The Elixir of Life," 182.
48 Margaret Sanger, *Woman and the New Race* (Brentano's, 1920), 178. See also: Carole Ruth McCann, *Birth Control Politics in the United States, 1916-1945* (Cornell University Press, 1994).
49 Nellie May Smith, *The Three Gifts of Life: A Girl's Responsibility for Race Progress* (Dodd, Mead and Company, 1913), 119.
50 Smith, *The Three Gifts of Life*, 105.
51 Smith, *The Three Gifts of Life*, 119-20.
52 Gilman, *The Crux*, 27.
53 Gilman, *The Crux*, 30.
54 Gilman, *The Crux*, 202.
55 Gilman, *The Crux*, 271.
56 Gilman, *The Crux*, 269.
57 Gilman, *The Crux*, 183.

58 Gilman, *The Crux*, 311.
59 Gilman, *The Crux*, 251.
60 Gilman, "Wild Oats and Tame Wheat," *The Forerunner* 4, no. 5 (1913), 130–31.
61 Gilman, "The Vintage," *The Forerunner* 7, no. 10 (1916), 253.
62 Gilman, "The Vintage," 254.
63 Gilman, "The Vintage," 254.
64 Gilman, "The Vintage," 257.
65 Paul A. Lombardo, "A Child's Right to Be Well Born: Venereal Disease and the Eugenic Marriage Laws, 1913–1935," *Perspectives in Biology and Medicine* 60, no. 2 (2017).
66 Hugh Cabot, "Syphilis and Society," *Social Hygiene* 2, no. 3 (1916), 347.
67 Cabot, "Syphilis and Society," 358.
68 Cabot, "Syphilis and Society," 347.
69 Gilman, "'The American Social Hygiene Association,' *Forerunner* 7, no. 9 (1916), 258.
70 Richard Cabot, "Are Sanitary Prophylaxis and Moral Prophylaxis Natural Allies?" *Journal of the Society of Sanitary and Moral Prophylaxis* 5, no. 1 (1914), 23.
71 Cabot, "Are Sanitary Prophylaxis and Moral Prophylaxis Natural Allies?" 21.
72 William J. Robinson, "Are Hygiene and Morality Natural Allies?" *The Medico-Pharmaceutical Critic and Guide* 17 (1914): 170.
73 Robinson, "Are Hygiene and Morality," 171.
74 Robinson, "Are Hygiene and Morality," 169.
75 Charlotte Perkins Gilman, "The Perpetuation of the Race," *Forerunner* 5, no. 7 (1914), 174.
76 Upton Sinclair, *Unseen Upton Sinclair: Nine Unpublished Stories, Essays and Other Works*, ed. Ruth Clifford Engs (McFarland, 2009).
77 Upton Sinclair, *Damaged Goods* (John C. Winston Company, 1913), 148.
78 Sinclair, *Damaged Goods*, 185.
79 Sinclair, *Damaged Goods*, 185.
80 Sinclair, *Damaged Goods*, 188.
81 Gilman, "Comment and Review," *The Forerunner* 4, no.4 (1913), 112.
82 1916–17 Upton Sinclair Letters to Frank Harris, Upton Sinclair Collection, Albert and Shirley Small Special Collections Library, University of Virginia.
83 Upton Sinclair, "Happy Marriage: How Can It Be Assured?" *Physical Culture* (1913), 299.
84 Sinclair, "Happy Marriage," 299.
85 Sinclair, "Happy Marriage," 298.
86 Sinclair, "Happy Marriage," 299.
87 Sinclair, "Happy Marriage," 300.
88 Sinclair, "Happy Marriage," 298.
89 Sinclair, *Sylvia's Marriage: a Novel* (Long Beach, 1914), 219.
90 Sinclair, *Sylvia's Marriage*, 219.
91 Sinclair, *Sylvia's Marriage*, 238.
92 Sinclair, *Sylvia's Marriage*, 238.
93 Sinclair, *Sylvia's Marriage*, 238.
94 Sinclair, *Sylvia's Marriage*, 252.
95 Sinclair, *Sylvia's Marriage*, 189.
96 Sinclair, *Sylvia's Marriage*, 11.
97 Sinclair, "Typescript of Early Draft," *Sylvia's Marriage*, box 23, Lilly Library, Indiana University, 2.

98 Sinclair, *Sylvia's Marriage*, 165.
99 Sinclair, *Sylvia's Marriage*, 166.
100 Sinclair, *Sylvia's Marriage*, 167.
101 Sinclair, *Sylvia's Marriage*, 167.
102 Sinclair, *Sylvia's Marriage*, 210.
103 Sinclair, *Sylvia's Marriage*, 254.
104 Sinclair, *Sylvia's Marriage*, 219.
105 Sinclair, *Sylvia's Marriage*, 239.
106 Sinclair, *Sylvia's Marriage*, 285.
107 Sinclair, *Sylvia's Marriage*, 285.
108 Sinclair, *Sylvia's Marriage*, 205.
109 Sinclair, *Sylvia's Marriage*, 95.
110 Sinclair, "Typescript of Early Draft," Upton Sinclair Papers, box 23, Lilly Library, Indiana University, 76.
111 Sinclair, *Sylvia's Marriage*, 93.
112 Sinclair, *Sylvia's Marriage*, 208.
113 Sinclair, *Sylvia's Marriage*, 210.
114 Sinclair, *Sylvia's Marriage*, 229.
115 Sinclair, *Sylvia's Marriage*, 286.
116 Robert N. Willson, "The Relation of the Medical Profession to the Social Evil," *Journal of the American Medical Association* 47, no. 1 (1906), 30.
117 Prince A. Morrow, "The Relations of Social Diseases to the Family," *American Journal of Sociology* 14, no. 5 (1909), 635.
118 Sinclair, *Sylvia's Marriage*, 287.
119 Russell H. Ramsey, "Report to Mr. Winston on 'Sylvia's Marriage,'" Upton Sinclair Papers, Lilly Library, Indiana University, 2–3.
120 Ramsey, "Report to Mr. Winston on 'Sylvia's Marriage,'" 1.
121 "The Problem Novel," *The Nation* 17 (August 1915), 716.
122 Sinclair, "The Profits of Religion," *A Monthly Magazine* 1, no 2. (1918).
123 Upton Sinclair, "Eugenic Celibate Motherhood," in *Unseen Upton Sinclair*, ed. Ruth Clifford Engs (McFarland, 2009), 98.
124 Sinclair, *The Book of Life, Volume II* (Haldeman-Julius Publications, 1921).
125 Sinclair, *The Book of Life, Volume II*, 83–4.
126 Sinclair, *The Book of Life, Volume II*, 84.
127 H. L. Mencken, *A Book of Burlesques* (John Lane Company, 1916).
128 Gilman, "Comment and Review," *Forerunner* 6, no. 3 (1915).

CHAPTER FOUR

1 As cited in Victor Robinson, "A Symposium on Euthanasia," *Medical Review of Reviews* 19 (1913), 152.
2 Jack London, "The Law of Life," *Children of the Frost* (Regent Press, 1913), 40.
3 Rosemarie Garland-Thomson, "The Cultural Logic of Euthanasia: 'Sad Fancyings' in Herman Melville's 'Bartleby,'" *American Literature* 76, no. 4 (2004), 783.
4 Shai Joshua Lavi, *The Modern Art of Dying: The History of Euthanasia in America* (Princeton University Press, 2005).
5 "Euthanasia," *Journal of the American Medical Association* XLI, no. 18 (1903).
6 Abraham Jacobi, "Euthanasia," *Medical Review of Reviews* 18, no. 6 (1912), 363.
7 Lavi, *Modern Art of Dying*, 109.

8   The original film (1916) was revised in 1927.
9   Martin S. Pernick, *The Black Stork: Eugenics and the Death of "Defective" Babies in American Medicine and Motion Pictures since 1915* (Oxford University Press, 1996), 5–6.
10 For a discussion of debilitating social conditions within liberal states, see Jasbir K. Puar, *The Right to Maim: Debility, Capacity, Disability* (Duke University Press, 2017).
11 Critics have only briefly discussed euthanasia in *The Monster* in terms of the intertwined forces of racism and ableism that Crane critiques. For instance, Susan Schweich cites the novella to illustrate how, in US culture, "race and disability are not separate but rather deeply associated and mutually reinforced," concerned as it is with "mercy killing." Price McMurray similarly points to the "central motive of the story, namely, the testing of the logic of racial euthanasia." Susan Schweik, "Disability Politics and American Literary History: Some Suggestions," American Literary History 20, no. 1/2 (2008). Price McMurray," Disabling Fictions: Race, History, and Ideology in Crane's 'The Monster,'" *Studies in American Fiction* 26, no. 1 (1998), 68.
12 Stephen Crane, *The Monster and Other Stories* (Harper, 1901), 3.
13 Gregory Laski accounts for this moment in terms of slavery, injury, and reparations. Gregory Laski, "'No Reparation': Accounting for the Enduring Harms of Slavery in Stephen Crane's *The Monster*," *J19* 1, no. 1 (2013).
14 Crane, *The Monster and Other Stories*, 28.
15 Crane, *The Monster and Other Stories*, 28–29.
16 Crane, *The Monster and Other Stories*, 44.
17 Crane, *The Monster and Other Stories*, 44.
18 Crane, *The Monster and Other Stories*, 45.
19 Martin S. Pernick, *The Black Stork: Eugenics and the Death of 'Defective' Babies in American Medicine and Motion Pictures Since 1915* (Oxford University Press, 1996), 90.
20 Crane, *The Monster and Other Stories*, 44.
21 Crane, *The Monster and Other Stories*, 46.
22 Crane, *The Monster and Other Stories*, 24.
23 Crane, *The Monster and Other Stories*, 30.
24 Crane, *The Monster and Other Stories*, 45.
25 Donald Pizer, "Stephen Crane's 'Maggie' and American Naturalism," *Criticism* 7, no. 2 (1965).
26 See, for instance, Ellen Samuels, *Fantasies of Identification: Disability, Gender, Race* (New York University Press, 2014).
27 Achille Mbembe, *Necropolitics* (Duke University Press, 2019).
28 Crane, *The Monster and Other Stories*, 39.
29 Crane, *The Monster and Other Stories*, 40.
30 Crane, *The Monster and Other Stories*, 41.
31 Crane, *The Monster and Other Stories*, 89.
32 Crane, *The Monster and Other Stories*, 66.
33 Crane, *The Monster and Other Stories*, 42.
34 Crane, *The Monster and Other Stories*, 98.
35 Crane, *The Monster and Other Stories*, 74.
36 Crane, *The Monster and Other Stories*, 74.

37 Edith Wharton to Sara Norton, June 3, 1901, Series II, box 29, folder 892, Edith Wharton Collection, Yale Collection of American Literature, Beinecke Rare Book and Manuscript Library.
38 Charles McGrath, "Wharton Letter Reopens a Mystery," *The New York Times*, November 1, 2007.
39 Edith Wharton to John Hugh Smith, Series II, box 26, folder 803, Edith Wharton Collection, Yale Collection of American Literature, Beinecke Rare Book and Manuscript Library.
40 Simeon Baldwin, "The Natural Right to a Natural Death," *Journal of Social Science* (December 1899).
41 Edith Wharton to Sara Norton, September 15, 1905, box 29, folder 899, Edith Wharton Collections, Yale Collection of American Literature, Beinecke Rare Book & Manuscript Library.
42 Edith Wharton to Sara Norton, July 7, 1908 in *The Letters of Edith Wharton*, ed. R.W.B. Lewis and Nancy Lewis (Scribner, 1988), 159, 163.
43 Jennie Kassanoff, *Edith Wharton and the Politics of Race* (Cambridge University Press, 2004).
44 Edith Wharton to Edward Burlingame, March 12, 1906, Scribner's Collection, Firestone Library, Princeton University.
45 Karen Weingarten, "Debility and Disability in Edith Wharton's Novels," *College Literature* 47, no. 3 (2020).
46 Edith Wharton, *The Fruit of the Tree* (Charles Scribner's Sons, 1907), 79.
47 Wharton, *Fruit of the Tree*, 69.
48 Wharton, *Fruit of the Tree*, 429.
49 Wharton, *Fruit of the Tree*, 11.
50 Jennie Kassanoff, "Corporate Thinking: Edith Wharton's *The Fruit of the Tree*," *Arizona Quarterly: A Journal of American Literature, Culture, and Theory* 53, no. 1 (1997).
51 Wharton, *Fruit of the Tree*, 15.
52 Wharton, *Fruit of the Tree*, 4.
53 James Tuttleton, "Justine; or, The Perils of Abstract Idealism," in *The Cambridge Companion to Edith Wharton*, ed. Millicent Bell (Cambridge University Press, 1995).
54 Wharton, *Fruit of the Tree*, 23.
55 Wharton, *Fruit of the Tree*, 58.
56 Wharton, *Fruit of the Tree*, 56–7.
57 Wharton, *Fruit of the Tree*, 56.
58 Wharton, *Fruit of the Tree*, 413.
59 Wharton, *Fruit of the Tree*, 431.
60 Wharton, *Fruit of the Tree*, 424.
61 Wharton, *Fruit of the Tree*, 433.
62 Rebecca Garden, "Sympathy, Disability, and the Nurse: Female Power in Edith Wharton's *The Fruit of the Tree*," *Journal of the Medical Humanities* 31, no. 3 (2010): 239.
63 Wharton, *Fruit of the Tree*, 526.
64 Wharton, *Fruit of the Tree*, 147.
65 Wharton, *Fruit of the Tree*, 525.
66 Wharton, *Fruit of the Tree*, 513.

67 Wharton, *Fruit of the Tree*, 585.
68 Wharton, *Fruit of the Tree*, 629.
69 Wharton, *Fruit of the Tree*, 146.
70 Wharton, *Fruit of the Tree*, 370.
71 Wharton, *Fruit of the Tree*, 413.
72 Wharton, *Fruit of the Tree*, 413.
73 Wharton, *Fruit of the Tree*, 588.
74 "Euthanasia as a Romantic Motive," *Journal of the American Medical Association* XLIX, no. 19 (1907), 1609.
75 "Euthanasia in Fiction: A Dangerous Misconception," *New York Medical Journal* 86 (November 2, 1907), 839.
76 Guy Flatley, "Thirty Years Later, Johnny Gets His Gun Again," *The New York Times*, June 28, 1970.
77 Dalton Trumbo to the Campbell, Silver, Cosby Corporation, "Is Johnny Too Extreme?," October 15, 1968, box 49, folder 1, Dalton Trumbo Papers, Charles E. Young Research Library, University of California, Los Angeles, 1–3.
78 Dalton Trumbo, *Johnny Got His Gun* (Citadel Press Books, 1939), 85.
79 Trumbo, *Johnny Got His Gun*, 232.
80 Trumbo, *Johnny Got His Gun*, 232.
81 Trumbo, *Johnny Got His Gun*, 231.
82 Trumbo, *Johnny Got His Gun*, 117.
83 Trumbo, *Johnny Got His Gun*, 114.
84 Trumbo, *Johnny Got His Gun*, 119.
85 Trumbo, *Johnny Got His Gun*, 83.
86 Trumbo, *Johnny Got His Gun*, 122.
87 Trumbo, *Johnny Got His Gun*, 88.
88 "Johnny Got His Gun by Dalton Trumbo, 3rd August 1939, Warner Brothers," box 1, folder 4, Dalton Trumbo Papers, The Wisconsin Center for Film and Theater Research, University of Wisconsin-Madison.
89 Trumbo, *Johnny Got His Gun*, 187.
90 Trumbo, *Johnny Got His Gun*, 180.
91 Trumbo, *Johnny Got His Gun*, 306.
92 Trumbo, *Johnny Got His Gun*, 306.
93 Dalton Trumbo to the Campbell, Silver, Cosby Corporation, June 26, 1968 box 49, folder 1, Dalton Trumbo Papers, Library Special Collections, Charles E. Young Research Library, University of California, Los Angeles, 3.
94 Trumbo to Kenneth Hyman, January 18, 1969, box 49, folder 1, Dalton Trumbo Papers, Charles E. Young Research Library, University of California, Los Angeles, 7.
95 Trumbo to Hyman, 7.
96 Trumbo to Hyman, 7.
97 Trumbo to Hyman, 7.
98 Trumbo to Hyman, 8–9.

CODA

1 Alondra Nelson, *Body and Soul: The Black Panther Party and the Fight Against Medical Discrimination* (University of Minnesota Press, 2011).
2 Eric Cassell, *The Place of the Humanities in Medicine* (The Hastings Center, 1984).
3 Cassell, *Place of the Humanities*, 7.

4 Cassell, *Place of the Humanities*, 13.
5 Ivan Illich, *Medical Nemesis: The Expropriation of Health* (Pantheon Books, 1976), 3.
6 Paul Starr, "The Politics of Therapeutic Nihilism," *The Hastings Center Report* 6, no. 5 (1976).
7 Michel Foucault, *The Birth of the Clinic: An Archaeology of Medical Perception*, trans. A. M. Sheridan (1963; Routledge, 1976).
8 Kathy Acker, "The Gift of Disease," *The Guardian*, Jan 8, 1997.
9 Boyer, *The Undying*, 169.
10 Boyer, *The Undying*, 195–96.
11 Leah Lakshmi Piepzna-Samarasinha, *Care Work: Dreaming Disability Justice* (Arsenal Pulp Press, 2018), 39.
12 Akemi Nishida, *Just Care: Messy Entanglements of Disability, Dependency, and Desire* (Temple University Press, 2022).
13 Johanna Hedva, "Sick Woman Theory," *Mask Magazine* 24 (2016).
14 Jonathan M. Metzl, "Introduction: Why Against Health?" in *Against Health: How Health Became the New Morality*, ed. Jonathan M. Metzl and Anna Kirkland (New York University Press, 2010), 1.
15 Lisa Howley, Elizabeth Gaufberg, and Brandy King, *The Fundamental Role of the Arts and Humanities in Medical Education* (Association of American Medical Colleges, 2020).
16 Craig M. Klugman and Erin Gentry Lamb, "Introduction: Raising Health Humanities," in *Research Methods in Health Humanities*, ed. Klugman and Lamb (Oxford University Press, 2019), 5.
17 Audre Lorde, *A Burst of Light and Other Essays* (Firebrand Books, 1988), 130.
18 Jina B. Kim and Sami Schalk, "Reclaiming the Radical Politics of Self-Care: A Crip-of-Color Critique," *The South Atlantic Quarterly* 120, no. 2 (2021), 329.
19 Lorde, *A Burst of Light*, 114.
20 Hiʻilei Julia Kawehipuaakahaopulani Hobart and Tamara Kneese, "Radical Care: Survival Strategies for Uncertain Times," *Social Text* 38, no. 1 (2020), 4.

Index

abortion, 23–24
access to medicine, 13–14, 25, 31, 35. *See also* charitable medical care
Acker, Kathy, 132–33, 136
African Americans: Black veterans' hospital, 56; hospitals and, 38–40, 49–50, 56–57; medical profession and, 37–39, 45, 47, 50, 52–56, 59; nursing and, 38–41, 48–49. *See also* psychiatry and race
The Age of Innocence (Wharton), 117
Ahad, Badia Sahar, 65
AIDS Coalition to Unleash Power, 130
alternative health and therapies: Christian Science, 51–52; health reform movements and, 3; homeopathy, 3–4; hydrotherapy, 4, 7; osteopathy, 6; self-care, 4, 37, 136–37; therapeutic nihilism, 2, 131–32, 135, 137
Altschuler, Sari, 11
American Medical Association (AMA), 5, 14, 28, 30
American Medicine Mobilizes (Rorty), 15
American Social Hygiene Association, 90
Archives of General Psychiatry, 66
Are You Fit to Marry (Haiselden, Lait), 109, 114
Arrow, Kenneth, 145n75
Arrowsmith (Lewis), 6
Asepsis (Mencken), 105
Association of American Medical Colleges, 5, 135

Baldwin, Simeon, 116
Barker, Lewellys F., 20
Barrish, Philip, 16
"Bartleby, the Scrivener" (Melville), 108
"Beating that Boy" (Ellison), 61
Beecher, Catherine, 79
Bellamy, Edward, 15
Bendiner, Robert, 68

Black Rage (Grier, Cobbs), 67, 69
Bollinger, Anna, 109
Bollinger, John, 109
Bonner, Marita, 36–38
Booker T. Washington Birthplace Memorial, 56
The Book of Life (Sinclair), 104–5
Boston Women's Health Book Collective, 130
Boyer, Anne, 133
Brieux, Eugene, 92
Bromberg, Walter, 66
Browner, Stephanie, 41
Bruce, La Marr Jurelle, 61
Burbick, Joan, 7
Burlingame, Edward, 116
A Burst of Light (Lorde), 136
Butler, Octavia, 73

Cabot, Hugh, 89–90
Cabot, Richard, 90–91
Campbell, J. Bradford, 61
Carnegie Foundation, 37
Cartwright, Samuel, 60
Cashman, Christopher R., 6
Cassell, Eric, 130–31
Cave, Henry W., 57
Chandler, Raymond, 13
charitable medical care, 14, 21, 25, 32, 35, 145n75
Charon, Rita, 11
Cheng, Anne Anlin, 65
Chesnutt, Charles Wadell: African American physicians and, 38, 42–43, 46–48, 52, 54, 59; critique of medical system, 37; cross-racial care, 9–10, 48; health and social protest, 1; nurse-patient relationship and, 39–41, 49, 53; politics and medicine, 45; racial injustices and, 72–73, 130; social protest of, 137

The Chicago Defender, 57–58
Claybaugh, Amanda, 8
Cobb, W. Montague, 55
Cobbs, Price M., 67, 69
commodification of medical care, 16–18
Comstock, Anthony, 75
Comstock Laws, 75
Concerning Children (Gilman), 81
conventional medicine, 6, 77, 132–33, 135
cost of care, 14, 17, 22, 27, 34
Council on Medical Education, 5
COVID-19 pandemic, 134–35
Cram, Ethel, 116
Crane, Stephen: on disability, 10, 126; on euthanasia, 109, 111–12, 114–15; health and social protest, 1; life and death questions, 110, 129; on medical autonomy, 130; naturalist characteristics of, 113; social protest of, 137
Crisis, 55
The Crux (Gilman), 10, 82–89, 92–93, 97, 103
The Custom of the Country (Wharton), 117
Cutter, Martha, 73, 84

Damaged Goods (Sinclair), 92–93, 95
Danielson, Susan, 41
Davis, Cynthia, 83
Davis, Harding, 14
de Kruif, Paul, 6
Derricotte, Juliette, 49–50
Dickinson, Emily, 7
Dingell, John D., 33
disability and disabled: characterization as dangerous, 114–15; collective care and, 134; distorted view of, 119; duty to die and, 126; medical profession and, 124–25, 130, 133; nature punishing of, 113; respect for, 127; stigmatization of, 10–11, 107, 110; value of, 123, 127; wounded soldiers, 123–24. *See also* euthanasia; *Johnny Got His Gun*
Dock, Lavinia, 81
The Doctor (Fildes), 30
Doty, Josh, 7
"Drab Rambles" (Bonner), 36–37
Dr. Kildare (Faust), 6
Du Bois, William Edward Burghardt, 52
duty to die, 10, 107, 110, 125–29

Ellison, Ralph: African American medical representation, 10; African American physicians and, 38; critique of medical system, 37; effect of anger, 69; effect of white hatred, 62–63; environment and mental health, 64–65; health and social protest, 1; mental illness diagnosis, 61; psychiatric racism, 71; psychiatry and, 59, 66; racial injustices and, 60, 67–68, 70, 72–73, 130
eugenics, 10, 77–78, 81–83, 85–88, 96, 98, 104
euthanasia: arguments for, 115, 120, 123; critical responses to, 10–11; definition of, 108; denunciation of, 109–10; disability and, 108–9, 111–13, 117, 128–29; exploitation of care, 119; legalization of, 116; London and, 107; medical professionalism and, 130; morphia-poisoning, 121; motives for, 118, 126–27; normalization of, 109; outside pressure and, 114; physician-assisted death, 108, 110, 115, 127–28. *See also The Fruit of the Tree*; "The Monster"
"Euthanasia as a Romantic Motive," 122
Evarts, Arrah B., 60
Eversley, Shelly, 60
Every Man His Own Doctor (Tennent), 2

Farm Security Administration, 14
Faust, Frederick Schiller, 6
Fildes, Luke, 30
The Fire in the Flint (White), 9, 50–55, 57–59, 73
Flexner, Abraham, 37
Folwell Stanford, Ann, 72–73
The Forerunner (Gilman), 80, 91
Frank, Arthur, 11
"free-floating hostility, 68–69
The Fruit of the Tree (Wharton), 11, 115–23, 126
Furman, A. I.: access to medicine, 14; cost of care and, 34; health and social protest, 1, 130; hospital corruption in, 9; institutional dysfunction and, 32; muckraking of, 21–22; profit-fueled and charitable care, 35; socioeconomic critique of medicine, 15, 23, 25

Gaines, Kevin, 42
Galton, Francis, 78
Garden, Rebecca, 120
Garland-Thomson, Rosemarie, 108
"Gift of Disease" (Acker), 132
gift of health, 15–21, 32, 35, 143n12
Gilman, Charlotte Perkins: on eugenics, 78; health and social protest, 1; marriage and depression, 84; on medical ethics, 85; on public health, 80, 86–87; sexual health advocacy, 10, 76, 81, 94, 103; on venereal disease, 77, 79, 83, 88–90, 92–93, 95, 104, 106, 130; white women's health and, 82; women's rights, 10, 91, 105
Gilman, Sander, 8
Golden Day pub (*Invisible Man*), 65–66, 68–72
Goldsby, Jacqueline, 112
Gordon, Linda, 82
Graham, Sylvester, 4
Gram, Hans Burch, 3
Grier, William H., 67, 69
Gulli, Andrew F., 13
Gunn, John C., 2

Haiselden, Harry, 109, 111–12
"Happy Marriage" (Sinclair), 94–96
Harlem Hospital, 56–57
"Harlem is Nowhere" (Ellison), 62–64, 67–69
The Healer (Herrick), 9, 16–21, 25, 32
Health Maintenance Organizations (HMO), 33–34
Hedva, Johanna, 134–36
Helen Brent, M. D. (Meyer), 74
Hernton, Calvin, 69
Herrick, Robert: access to medicine, 14; capitalism and medical care, 16–17, 19–21; cost of care and, 34; gift economy, 18, 32; health and social protest, 1, 130; socioeconomic critique of medicine, 9, 15; state funded medicine, 25
Hobart, Hi'ilei Julia Kawehipuaakahaopulani, 136
Hoeller, Hildegard, 143n12
Holmes, Oliver Wendell Sr., 7
Home of the Brave (film), 64

hospitals, inequalities of, 21–22
The House of Mirth (Wharton), 115, 117
Hughes, Langston, 21
Hylan, John F., 56

"The Ideal Nurse" (Chesnutt), 38, 41, 47–49, 53
Illich, Ivan, 132
The Interne (Furman, Thurman), 9, 21–25, 32
Invisible Man (Ellison), 10, 59–61, 65–73
"It's All Right—He Only Died" (Chandler), 13

Jacobi, Abraham, 109
Johnny Got His Gun (film), 126–28
Johnny Got His Gun (Trumbo), 11, 123–29
Journal of the American Medical Association, 20, 32, 109, 122
The Jungle (Sinclair), 20, 92
Jurecic, Ann, 11

Karpman, Benjamin, 67
Kassanoff, Jennie, 118
Keller, Helen, 109
Kim, Jina B., 136
Kinnicutt, Francis, 115
"Kitchen-Mindedness" (Gilman), 79
Klugman, Craig, 136
Knadler, Stephen, 42
Kneese, Tamara, 136–37
Koch, Robert, 5
Kuhn, Hartmann, 116

Lafargue, Paul, 60
Lafargue Mental Hygienic Clinic, 10, 60–64, 68
Lait, Jack, 109
Lamb, Erin, 136
"The Law of Life" (London), 107, 113
Les Avariés (Brieux), 92
Lewis, Robert, 112
Lewis, R. W. B., 117
Lewis, Sinclair, 6
"Life in the Iron Mills" (Davis), 14–15
London, Jack, 107, 113, 133
Looking Backward (Bellamy), 15
Lorde, Audre, 136

Magazine of the Year, 69
Maggie (Crane), 113
A Man Called White (White), 56
Manly Health and Training (Whitman), 3
The Marrow of Tradition (Chesnutt), 9, 41–49, 52–54, 73, 137
Marx, Leo, 17–18
McMurray, Price, 154n11
"Medical Care and the Plight of the Negro," (Cobb), 55
medical humanities, 11, 130–32, 136
medical-industrial complex, 32, 130, 132
Medical Nemesis (Illich), 132
medical professionalism, 11, 28, 41–48, 50–52, 72–73, 85, 88, 97, 120, 130, 132, 135
Medical Review of Reviews, 93, 107
Melville, Herman, 7, 108
Mencken, H. L., 105
Metzl, Jonathan, 66, 135
Meyer, Annie Nathan, 74–76
Microbe Hunters (de Kruif), 6
Mitchell, Silas Weir, 79
The Monster (Crane), 10, 110–15, 118, 126, 137, 154n11
A Monthly Magazine, 103
Morris, Robert, 6
Morrison, Toni, 73
Morrow, Prince A., 76, 81, 84, 90, 94, 102, 104
Morse, Wayne, 56
muckraking, 16, 21–22, 92–93
Murray, James E., 33

The Nation, 103
National Association for the Advancement of Colored People (NAACP), 9, 49, 55, 57
national health insurance, 9, 14, 25–26, 28, 34
Native Son (R. Wright), 67
naturalism, 107, 113
"The Natural Right to a Natural Death" (Baldwin), 116
Negro Year Book, 40
Never-Told Tales (Robinson), 78
Nevius, Blake, 18
New Guide to Health (Thomson), 3
New York Herald Tribune, 55

New York Medical Journal, 122
The New York Times, 6, 13, 123
Nichols, Mary Sargeant Gove, 4
Nightingale, Florence, 38
Nishida, Akemi, 134
North Harlem Medical Association, 56–57
Norton, Charles, 116
Norton, Sara "Sally," 115–16
No Way Out (film), 58–59

Oppenheim, James, 74–76
Our Bodies, Ourselves, 130

"The Paid Nurse" (Williams), 15
Pasteur, Louis, 5
patriarchal society and attitudes, 75–79, 81, 85, 87–89, 93, 97–99, 101, 106
Physical Culture, 94, 96, 98, 102
Piepzna-Samarasinha, Lakshmi, 133–34
Pittman, Portia Washington, 56
The Place of the Humanities in Medicine (Cassell), 131
Poe, Edgar Allan, 7
Poitier, Sidney, 58
"The 'Protest' Psychosis" (Bromberg, Simon), 66
psychiatry and race, 59–70, 72–73
The Psychoanalytical Review, 60
public health, 1, 10, 77, 79–83, 85–89, 91–93, 106, 134–35. *See also* venereal disease
public hospitals, 15, 21–25

racial justice and racism, 36–39, 41–43, 45, 49–55, 62, 72–73, 130. *See also* African Americans; eugenics
"Remarks on Osteopathy" (Twain), 6
"Richard Wright's Blues" (Ellison), 62
right to die, 10, 107–10, 116, 120, 123, 125, 129
Robinson, William J., 78–80, 90–91
Roosevelt, Eleanor, 57
Roosevelt, Franklin Delano, 14
Roosevelt, Theodore, 14
Rorty, James, 15
Russell, Stephen, 133

Sanger, Margaret, 85–86
Scarecrow, Scarecrow (Hernton), 69

Schalk, Sami, 136
Schweich, Susan, 154n11
sexual morality, 77–78, 88, 90
"The Shadow and the Act" (Ellison), 64–65
"Sick Woman Theory" (Hedva), 134
Simon, Franck, 66
Sinclair, Mary Craig, 92
Sinclair, Upton: comparison to Herrick, 20; culture of prudery, 95; on eugenics, 78; health and social protest, 1; patriarchal culture of medicine and, 98; sexual health advocacy, 10, 76, 92; social protest of, 137; on venereal disease, 96–97, 100–106, 130; white women's health and, 93; women's health and, 94, 99; women's rights, 10
Slaughter, Frank: access to medical care, 14, 25, 31, 35; background of, 26; cost of care and, 34; descriptions of healing, 27; doctor-patient relationship and, 32; health and social protest, 1, 130; national health insurance and, 9, 28–30, 33; socioeconomic critique of medicine, 15
Smith, Cera, 61
Smith, John Hugh, 116
Smith, Nellie May, 86
Social Diseases and Marriage (Morrow), 81
socialist medicine and socialism, 9, 20, 28–31, 33, 35
social realism, 8
Society of Moral Prophylaxis, 76, 82, 86, 90–91
Sontag, Susan, 7
Southern Medical Association, 55
Starr, Paul, 2, 131
Stetson, Walter, 83
Strand Magazine, 13
Sweeney, Brian, 42
Sylvia's Marriage (Sinclair), 10, 92, 95–103, 105–6, 137

Tavera, Stephanie Peebles, 77
Tennent, John, 2
That None Should Die (Slaughter), 9, 25–34
Thomson, Samuel, 3
Thomsonianism, 3

The Three Gifts of Life (Smith), 86
Thurman, Wallace: access to medicine, 14; cost of care and, 34; health and social protest, 1, 130; hospital corruption in, 9; institutional dysfunction and, 32; muckraking of, 21–22; profit-fueled and charitable care, 35; socioeconomic critique of medicine, 15, 23, 25
Tomes, Nancy, 2
A Treatise on Domestic Economy (Beecher), 79
Truman, Harry, 14, 30, 33
Trumbo, Dalton: on disability, 10–11, 130; disabled veterans and, 123–25; duty to die and, 126–27; on euthanasia, 109, 128; health and social protest, 1; life and death questions, 129
Twain, Mark, 6

The Undying (Boyer), 133

Velsor, Mose. *See* Whitman, Walt
venereal disease: American Plan, 75–76; attitudes toward, 88; Comstock Laws and, 75, 95; confidentiality and, 84–85, 89; control of, 76–79, 91–92, 94; definition of, 150n2; disclosure of, 89, 95; effect on women, 82; knowledge and understanding of, 99–101, 103–4; marriage and, 98, 102; medical certificate to marry, 83; medical theories of, 10; Mencken's satire and, 105; numbers of cases, 101, 104; public reporting of, 89–90; secrecy around, 74–75, 80–81, 89, 94, 96–97, 100, 130; transmission and blame, 93, 103; treatments, 77, 86, 90
"The Vintage" (Gilman), 88–89

Wagner, Robert F., 33
Wagner-Murray-Dingell bill, 33
Wald, Lillian, 109
Warren Plan, 26, 31–34
The Web of Life (Herrick), 16
Weingarten, Karen, 24, 117
Weinstein, Cindy, 84
Wertham, Frederic, 60, 68
Wharton, Edith: on disability, 10; on euthanasia, 11, 109, 115–17, 122–23, 126;

Wharton, Edith: (*continued*):
    health and social protest, 1; industrial capitalism and, 118–19; life and death questions, 129; nurse-patient relationship and, 120; on nursing, 121; respect for life, 130
White, George (Walter's father), 49–50, 58
White, Walter: African American medical representation, 10; African American physicians and, 38, 51, 54; Black veterans' hospital and, 56; critique of medical system, 37; desegregation of medicine, 9, 49, 55, 57, 59; health and social protest, 1; his father's death and, 50, 58; racial injustices and, 72–73, 130; racial violence and, 52; white supremacism and, 53
Whitman, Walt, 3, 7
Wild Oats (Oppenheim), 74–75, 81
"Wild Oats and Tame Wheat" (Gilman), 88

Williams, Andreá N., 42
Williams, Williams Carlos, 6, 15
Willson, Robert, 101–2
Woman and the New Race (Sanger), 85
Women and Economics (Gilman), 80
women's health, 102; divorce and separation and, 78, 84, 94–95, 101–2, 104; marriage and, 94–95, 105; men's wild oats and sexual desires, 75, 77, 87–88, 91–92, 99, 103–4; prostitution and, 77, 93–94, 104, 113; sex education and, 74, 77, 82, 89, 91, 101; sexual autonomy, 77, 86; silence and secrecy, 74; sterilization and, 78, 98. *See also* venereal disease
Woodhull, Victoria, 85
Wright, Louis, 56–57
Wright, Richard, 60, 67

"The Yellow Wall-Paper" (Gilman), 79

Ziegler, Mary, 82

www.ingramcontent.com/pod-product-compliance
Lightning Source LLC
Chambersburg PA
CBHW021624250426
43672CB00037B/2566